50 STUDIES EVERY DOCTOR SHOULD KNOW

The Key Studies that Form the Foundation of Evidence Based Medicine

D1314254

MICHAEL E. HOCHMAN, MD

ISBN: 1469975998
ISBN 13: 9781469975993

ABOUT THE AUTHOR

Dr. Michael Hochman is a board certified general internist who attended Princeton University and Harvard Medical School. He completed his residency in internal medicine at the Cambridge Health Alliance in Cambridge, Massachusetts. Following residency, Dr. Hochman worked as an attending physician at the Keck School of Medicine of the University of Southern California and the Los Angeles County + University of Southern California Medical Center. Currently, Dr. Hochman is a fellow in the *Robert Wood Johnson Foundation Clinical Scholars* program at the University of California, Los Angeles, with support from the U.S. Department of Veterans Affairs.

Dr. Hochman has an interest in communicating complex medical information in a digestible format. He has written numerous medically related articles for the *Boston Globe* and other lay media publications. In addition, Dr. Hochman enjoys teaching and has won several clinical teaching awards. Dr. Hochman has also published original research in top medical journals including the *Journal of the American Medical Association.*

DEDICATION

This book is dedicated to my family – mom, Steve, Jess, and Emma.

INTERESTED IN WRITING?

I hope to develop an evidence-based medicine series covering all of the medical specialties, e.g. "50 Studies Every Psychiatrist Should Know", "50 Studies Every Cardiologist Should Know" etc. If you are interested in writing a book in this series, e-mail me at: meh1979@gmail.com.

TABLE OF CONTENTS

Section 3: Surgery

Section 4: Obstetrics

Section 5: Pediatrics

Section 6: Radiology

Section 7: Neurology and Psychiatry

Section 8: Systems Based Practice

PREFACE

When I was a third year medical student, I asked one of my senior residents – who seemed to be able to quote every medical study in the history of mankind – if he had a list of key studies I should read before graduating medical school. "Don't worry," he told me. "You will learn the key studies as you go along."

But picking up on these key studies didn't prove so easy for me and I was frequently admonished by my attendings for being unaware of well-known studies. More importantly, because I had a mediocre understanding of the medical literature, I lacked confidence in my clinical decision-making and had difficulty appreciating the significance of new research findings. It wasn't until I was well into my residency – and after considerable effort – that I finally began to feel comfortable with the medical literature.

Now, as a practicing general internist, I realize that I am not the only doctor who has struggled to become familiar with the key medical studies that form the foundation of evidence based practice. Many of the students and residents I work with tell me that they feel overwhelmed by the medical literature, and that they cannot process new research findings because they lack a solid understanding of what has already been published. In addition, I have found that many practicing physicians – including some with years of experience – have only a cursory knowledge of the medical literature and base clinical decisions largely on personal experience rather than evidence.

I have written this book – a compilation of summaries of "50 studies every doctor should know" – in an attempt to provide medical professionals (and even lay readers interested in learning more about medical research) a quick way to get up-to-speed on the classic studies that shape clinical practice. In addition, I have provided a case at the end of each study so that readers can practice applying research findings to clinical decision-making (after all, it is not good enough just to know the key studies, you also must also be able to apply the findings in real-world situations). I have tried to present the studies in a simple and engaging way, highlighting the critical points and removing the unnecessary jargon. As you read through the summaries, I hope you will realize that medical research is not as intimidating as it might initially seem.

You may be wondering how I selected the 50 studies I included in this book. There are, of course, no perfect criteria for making such selections. In the end, I opted to include the studies I have personally found to be most influential and that address areas of controversy in medicine. In many cases, I also consulted my colleagues for suggestions. I hope to receive feedback from readers about which studies to include in future editions of this book.

Finally, a note about how this book was published: when I initially proposed this book to several traditional medical publishing companies, most were interested. However, they all told me that I would need to double the size so that they could "justify" charging over $100 – the minimum price that is needed for most medical textbooks like this to be profitable. Not only did I think that doubling the size could be overwhelming to readers, but the high cost was not consistent with my mission of writing a book that would be affordable for a wide audience of readers. In the end, I decided to self-publish the book through CreateSpace (a popular self-publishing company) so that I would have more control over the content and price. Because I did not have a professional editor, I asked the authors of studies included in this book to review my summaries for accuracy and 90% complied.

I hope you enjoy reading about these key medical studies, and that this book will serve as a building block for understanding and practicing evidence based medicine!

– Michael Hochman, MD

ACKNOWLEDGMENTS

Thanks goes to Dr. Carlos Lerner and Dr. Jessica Matthew Hochman (my wife) for assistance writing the Pediatrics section of this book.

In addition, I would like to acknowledge the *Robert Wood Johnson Foundation Clinical Scholars* program in which I was a fellow while writing this book, as well as Dr. Ken Wells from the *Clinical Scholars* program for his advice and support.

I would also like to thank the medical students and residents at the Cambridge Health Alliance and the Los Angeles County + University of Southern California Medical Center, particularly Dr. Behzad Yashar, for encouraging me to write this book.

Finally, I would like to thank the 45 authors of studies included in this book who graciously reviewed my summaries for accuracy (43 of their names are listed below, and two authors asked to remain anonymous). I very much appreciate the assistance of these authors. Importantly, however, the views expressed in this book do not represent those of the authors acknowledged below, nor do these authors vouch for the accuracy of the information; any mistakes are my own.

Michael Hochman, MD

- Dr. William C. Knowler, Diabetes Prevention Program Writing Committee for: Reduction in the incidence of type 2 diabetes with lifestyle intervention or metformin. N Engl J Med. 2002 Feb 7;346(6):393-403.

- Dr. Frank M. Sacks, first author of: Comparison of weight-loss diets with different compositions of fat, protein, and carbohydrates. N Engl J Med. 2009;360:859-73.

- Dr. Charles H. Hennekens, Principle Investigator of the Physicians' Health Study Research Group and Chairman of the Steering Committee for: Final report on the aspirin component of the ongoing Physicians' Health Study. N Engl J Med. 1989 Jul 20;321(3):129-35.

- Dr. Paul M. Ridker, first author of: A randomized trial of low-dose aspirin in the primary prevention of cardiovascular disease in women. N Engl J Med. 2005 Mar 31;352(13):1293-304.

- Dr. Rowan T. Chlebowski, member of the Women's Health Initiative Steering Committee for: Risks and benefits of estrogen plus progestin in healthy postmenopausal women: principal results from the Women's Health Initiative randomized controlled trial. JAMA. 2002 Jul 17;288(3):321-33.

- Dr. Fritz H. Schröder, first author of: Prostate-cancer mortality at 11 years of follow-up. N Engl J Med. 2012 Mar 15;366(11):981-90.

- Dr. Debra S. Echt, first author of: Mortality and morbidity in patients receiving encainide, flecainide, or placebo. N Engl J Med. 1991 Mar 21;324(12):781-788.

- Dr. William C. Cushman, member of the ALLHAT Group Steering Committee for: Major outcomes in high-risk hypertensive patients randomized to angiotensin-converting enzyme inhibitor or calcium channel blocker vs diuretic: The antihypertensive and lipid-lowering treatment to prevent heart attack trial (ALLHAT). JAMA. 2002 Dec 18;288(23):2981-97.

- Dr. Paul M. Ridker, Principle Investigator, Trial Chair, and first author of: Rosuvastatin to prevent vascular events in men and women with elevated C-reactive protein. N Engl J Med. 2008 Nov 20;359(21):2195-2207.

- Dr. Brian Olshanksy, member of the AFFIRM investigators for: A comparison of rate control and rhythm control in patients with atrial fibrillation. N Engl J Med. 2002 Dec 5;347(23):1825-33.

- Dr. Isabelle C. Van Gelder, Chair of the Writing Committee and Chair of the Steering Committee for the RACE II Study Group, and first author of: Lenient vs. strict rate control in patients with atrial fibrillation. N Engl J Med. 2010 Apr 15;362(15):1363-73.

- Dr. John Wikstrand, co-author of: Effects of controlled-release metoprolol on total mortality, hospitalizations, and well-being in patients with heart failure: The metoprolol CR/XL randomized intervention trial in congestive heart failure. JAMA. 2000;283(10):1295-1302.

- Dr. William E. Boden, co-chair for the COURAGE Trial Research Group, and first author of: Optimal medical therapy with or without PCI for stable coronary disease. N Engl J Med. 2007 Apr 12;356(15):1503-16.

- Dr. Anne L. Taylor, Chair of the A-HeFT Steering Committee and first author of: Combination of isosorbide dinitrate and hydralazine in blacks with heart failure. N Engl J Med. 2004 Nov 11;351(20):2049-2056.

- Dr. Emanuel Rivers, first author of: Early goal-directed therapy in the treatment of severe sepsis and septic shock. N Engl J Med. 2001 Nov 8;345(19):1368-77.

- Dr. Paul C. Hébert, first author of: A multicenter, randomized, controlled clinical trial of transfusion requirements in critical care. N Engl J Med. 1999 Feb 11;340(6):409-17.

- Dr. Christian Richard, first author of: Early use of the pulmonary artery catheter and outcomes in patients with shock and acute respiratory distress syndrome. JAMA. 2003 Nov 26;290(20):2713-2720.

- Corine van Marrewijk, first author of: Effect and cost-effectiveness of step-up vs. step-down treatment with antacids, H2-receptor antagonists, and proton pump inhibitors in patients with new onset dyspepsia (DIAMOND study): a primary-care-based randomized controlled trial. The Lancet. 2009 Jan 17;373:215-225.

- Dr. Dwight E. Moulin, first author of: Randomised trial of oral morphine for chronic non-cancer pain. Lancet. 1996;347:143-147.

- Dr. Philip J. Devereaux, first author of: Effects of extended-release metoprolol succinate in patients undergoing non-cardiac surgery (POISE trial): a randomised controlled trial. Lancet. 2008 May 31;371(9627):1839-47.

- Dr. Patrick W. Serruys, first author of: Percutaneous coronary intervention vs. coronary-artery bypass grafting for severe coronary artery disease. N Engl J Med. 2009 Mar 5;360(10):961-972.

- Professor Alison Halliday, Principle Investigator for the MRC Asymptomatic Carotid Surgery Trial (ACST) Collaborative Group and first author of: Prevention of disabling and fatal strokes by successful carotid endarterectomy in patients without recent neurological symptoms: randomized controlled trial. Lancet. 2004 May 8;363(9420):1491-502.

- Dr. Robert B. Litchfield, co-author of: A randomized trial of arthroscopic surgery for osteoarthritis of the knee. N Engl J Med. 2008 Sep 11;359(11):1097-107.

- Professor Jeremy Fairbank, first author of: Randomised controlled trial to compare surgical stabilization of the lumbar spine with an intensive rehabilitation programme for patients with chronic lower back pain: the MRC spine stabilisation trial. BMJ. 2005 May 28;330(7502):1233.

- Dr. Bernard Fisher, first author of: Twenty-year follow-up of a randomized trial comparing total mastectomy, lumpectomy, and lumpectomy plus irradiation for the treatment of invasive breast cancer. N Engl J Med. 2002 Oct 17;347(16):1233-1241.

- Dr. Lars Sjöström, first author of: Effects of bariatric surgery on mortality in Swedish obese subjects. N Engl J Med. 2007 Aug 23;357(8):741-52.

- Dr. Alejandro Hoberman, first author of: Treatment of acute otitis media in children under 2 years of age. N Engl J Med. 2011; 364(2):105-115.

- Dr. Jack L. Paradise, first author of: Effect of early or delayed insertion of tympanostomy tubes for persistent otitis media on developmental outcomes at the age of three years. N Engl J Med. 2001 Apr 19;344(16):1179-1187.

- Dr. Paul M. O'Byrne, co-author of: Early intervention with budesonide in mild persistent asthma: a randomized, double-blind trial. Lancet. 2003 Mar 29;361:1071-1076.

- Dr. Peter S. Jensen, a Principal Collaborator for the Multimodal Treatment Study of Children With Attention-Deficit/Hyperactivity Disorder Cooperative Group and the corresponding author for: A 14-month randomized clinical trial of treatment strategies for attention-deficit/hyperactivity disorder. Arch Gen Psychiatry. 1999;56:1073-1086.

- Dr. Kreesten Meldgaard Madsen, first author of: A population-based study of measles, mumps, and rubella vaccination and autism. N Engl J Med. 2002 Nov 347;19: 1477-1482.

- Dr. Jeffrey (Jerry) G. Jarvik, first author of: Rapid magnetic resonance imaging vs radiographs for patients with low back pain: a randomized controlled trial. JAMA. 2003;289(21):2810-2718.

ACKNOWLEDGMENTS

- Dr. Frans J Th Wackers, Principal Investigator and Chair of DIAD and senior author of: Cardiac outcomes after screening for asymptomatic coronary artery disease in patients with type 2 diabetes: the DIAD study: a randomized controlled trial. JAMA. 2009 Apr 15;301(15):1547-55.

- Dr. Menno V. Huisman, corresponding author of: Effectiveness of managing suspected pulmonary embolism using an algorithm combining clinical probability, D-dimer testing, and computed tomography. JAMA. 2006 Jan 11;295(2):172-9.

- Dr. Nathan Kuppermann, first author of: Identification of children at very low risk of clinically-important brain injuries after head trauma: a prospective cohort study. The Lancet. 2009;374:1160-1170.

- Dr. Werner Hacke, Chair of the Steering Committee for the European Cooperative Acute Stroke Study (ECASS) and first author of: Thrombolysis with alteplase 3 to 4.5 hours after acute ischemic stroke. NEJM. 2008 Sep 25;359(13):1317-1329.

- Dr. Herbert C. Schulberg, first author of: Treating major depression in primary care practice. Arch Gen Psychiatry. 1996;53:913-919.

- Dr. Charles M. Morin, first author of: Behavioral and pharmacological therapies for late-life insomnia: A randomized controlled trial. JAMA. 1999;281(11):991-999.

- Dr. Robert Reid, first author of: The Group Health medical home at year two: cost savings, higher patient satisfaction, and less burnout for providers. Health Aff (Millwood). 2010 May;29(5):835-43.

- Dr. Brian Jack, first author of: A reengineered hospital discharge program to decrease rehospitalization. Annals of Internal Medicine. 2009;150:178-187.

- Dr. Peter Pronovost, first author of: An intervention to decrease catheter-related bloodstream infections in the ICU. N Engl J Med. 2006 Dec 28;355(26):2725-32.

- Dr. Jennifer S. Temel, first author of: Early palliative care for patients with metastatic non-small-cell lung cancer. N Engl J Med. 2010 Aug 19;363(8):733-42.

- Dr. C. Patrick Chaulk, first author of: Eleven years of community-based directly observed therapy for tuberculosis. JAMA. 1995;274:945-951.

SECTION 1:

PREVENTIVE MEDICINE

PREVENTING DIABETES:

THE DIABETES PREVENTION PROGRAM[1]

"Our study showed that treatment with metformin and modification of lifestyle were two highly effective means of delaying or preventing type 2 diabetes. The lifestyle intervention was particularly effective, with one case of diabetes prevented per seven persons treated for three years."

— The Diabetes Prevention Program Research Group[1]

Research Question: Can the onset of type 2 diabetes be prevented or delayed with metformin and/or lifestyle modifications?

Funding: The National Institutes of Health, the Indian Health Service, the Centers for Disease Control and Prevention, the General Clinical Research Center Program, the American Diabetes Association, Bristol-Myers Squibb, and Parke-Davis Pharmaceuticals.

Year Study Began: 1996

Year Study Published: 2002

Study Location: 27 clinical centers in the U.S.

---

1 Diabetes Prevention Program Research Group. Reduction in the incidence of type 2 diabetes with lifestyle intervention or metformin. N Engl J Med. 2002 Feb 7;346(6):393-403.

Who Was Studied: Adults ≥25 years old with a body-mass index (BMI) ≥24 kg/m², a fasting plasma glucose of 95-125 mg/dl, and a plasma glucose of 140-199 mg/dl two hours after a 75-g oral glucose load.

Who Was Excluded: People with diagnosed diabetes, those taking medications known to alter glucose tolerance, and those with serious illnesses that could reduce life expectancy or interfere with the ability to participate in the trial.

How Many Participants: 3,234

Study Overview:

Figure 1: Summary of the Trial's Design

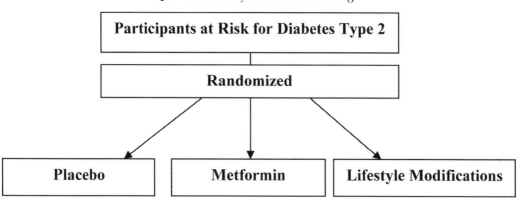

Study Interventions: Participants in the placebo group received standard lifestyle recommendations. Participants in the metformin group received standard lifestyle recommendations along with metformin 850 mg twice daily. Participants in the lifestyle group were given an intensive lifestyle modification program taught by case managers on a one-to-one basis with the goal of achieving and maintaining a 7% or greater reduction in body weight, improvements in dietary intake, and physical activity of at least 150 minutes per week. The lifestyle modification program was taught during 16 sessions over a 24-week period, and reinforced with individual (usually monthly) and group sessions after that.

Follow-Up: Mean of 2.8 years

Endpoint: Primary outcome: Diabetes, as defined by either a fasting glucose ≥126 mg/dl or a glucose ≥200 two hours after a 75-g oral glucose load on two separate occasions.

RESULTS:

- the average participant in the lifestyle group lost 5.6 kg during the study period vs. 2.1 kg in the metformin group and 0.1 kg in the placebo group (P<0.001)

- participants in the lifestyle group reported significantly more physical activity than those in the metformin and placebo groups, and at the final study visit 58% reported at least 150 minutes per week of physical activity

- participants in the metformin group had approximately six times the rate of gastrointestinal symptoms as participants in the lifestyle group, while the rate of musculoskeletal symptoms was approximately 1.2 times higher among participants in the lifestyle group compared with those in the metformin group

Table 1: Estimated Cumulative Incidence of Diabetes at 3 Years

Placebo	Metformin	Lifestyle Modifcations
28.9%[a]	21.7%[a]	14.4%[a]

[a]Differences all statistically significant

Criticisms and Limitations: The participants assigned to the lifestyle group achieved an impressive reduction in weight, as well as impressive improvements in dietary and exercise patterns. This suggests that study participants were highly motivated individuals. Such successes might not be possible in other populations. In addition, the trial did not assess whether either the lifestyle intervention or metformin led to a reduction in hard clinical endpoints, such as diabetes-related microvascular disease.

Other Relevant Studies and Information:

- A recently published 10-year follow-up evaluation of participants in the Diabetes Prevention Program showed that the cumulative incidence of diabetes remained 34% lower in the lifestyle group and 18% lower in the metformin group compared to the placebo group[2].

---

2 Diabetes Prevention Program Research Group. 10-year follow-up of diabetes incidence and weight loss in the diabetes prevention program outcomes study. Lancet. 2009 Nov 14;374(9702):1677-86..

SUMMARY AND IMPLICATIONS:

To prevent one case of diabetes over three years, approximately 7 people must be treated with a lifestyle-intervention program or approximately 14 must be treated with metformin. Lifestyle modifications are, therefore, the preferred method for preventing or delaying the onset of diabetes.

CLINICAL CASE: PREVENTING DIABETES

CASE HISTORY:

A 54 year old woman is found to have pre-diabetes with a fasting plasma glucose of 116 on two separate occasions. She is overweight with a BMI of 29, and reports only very limited physical activity.

As this woman's doctor, you recommend that she begin a weight-loss and exercise program to reduce her risk for developing diabetes. But she is hesitant, and tells you she is too busy to make lifestyle changes. In addition, "none of this lifestyle stuff works anyway."

Based on the results of the Diabetes Prevention Program, what can you tell your patient about the potential impact of lifestyle changes for preventing diabetes?

SUGGESTED ANSWER:

The Diabetes Prevention Program unequivocally demonstrated that lifestyle modifications – more so than medications – can reduce the risk of developing diabetes. Thus, you can tell your patient that there is good evidence from a well designed study that lifestyle changes can work.

Since this woman is busy and may not have the time to participate in an intensive program like the study participants in the Diabetes Prevention Program did, you might give her some simple recommendations she can follow on her own, for example walking for 30 minutes a day. You might also give her manageable goals, for example a 5-10 pound weight loss at her next visit with you in three months.

A COMPARISON OF DIFFERENT DIETING STRATEGIES[3]

"[A]ny type of diet, when taught for the purpose of weight loss with enthusiasm and persistence, can be effective ... the specific [type of diet] is of minor importance ..."

- Sacks et al.[3]

Research Question: Which type of diet is best: a low fat diet, a low protein diet, or a low carbohydrate diet?

Funding: The National Heart, Lung, and Blood Institute and the General Clinical Research Center, National Institutes of Health.

Year Study Began: 2004

Year Study Published: 2009

---

3 Sacks et al. Comparison of weight-loss diets with different compositions of fat, protein, and carbohydrates. NEJM. 2009;360:859-73.

Study Location: The Harvard School of Public Health and Brigham and Women's Hospital in Boston, and the Pennington Biomedical Research Center, Louisiana State University.

Who Was Studied: Adults 30-70 with a body-mass index (BMI) of 25-40 who were recruited with mass mailings.

Who Was Excluded: Patients with diabetes, unstable cardiovascular disease, patients taking medications affecting body weight, and those with "insufficient motivation as assessed by interview and questionnaire."

How Many Patients: 811

Study Overview:

Figure 1: Summary of the Trial's Design

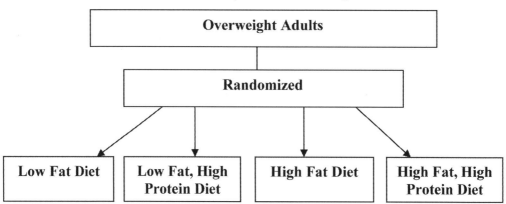

Study Intervention: Patients in all four groups received regular group sessions for nutritional and behavioral counseling. For the first six months, sessions were held 3 out of every 4 weeks, and from six months to two years the sessions were held 2 out of every 4 weeks. In addition, patients received individual sessions every eight weeks for the entire two years.

Patients assigned to each group attended separate sessions but were not told which diet they had been assigned to. Instead, they were given recommended meal plans that were consistent with their assigned diet. Each meal plan was individualized and recommended 750 fewer calories than each patient's baseline food intake.

The four diets were designed as follows:

- **Low Fat:** 20% fat, 15% protein, and 65% carbohydrates
- **Low Fat, High Protein:** 20% fat, 25% protein, and 55% carbohydrates

- **High Fat:** 40% fat, 15% protein, and 45% carbohydrates

- **High Fat, High Protein:** 40% fat, 25% protein, and 35% carbohydrates

In addition, all four diets recommended ≤8% saturated fat intake, ≥20 grams of dietary fiber intake, a low cholesterol content, and carbohydrates with a low glycemic index.

Follow-Up: Two years

Endpoints: Primary outcome: Change in body weight over two years. Secondary outcomes: Changes in waist circumference; changes in low-density lipoprotein (LDL) and high-density lipoprotein (HDL) levels; changes in blood pressure; changes in the prevalence of the metabolic syndrome; and satisfaction with the diet.

RESULTS:

- Among patients who completed the study, the mean age was 52, the mean BMI was 33, and 36% had hypertension

- Most of the weight loss among study patients occurred in the first 6 months of the dieting period

Table 1: Weight Loss with Different Dieting Strategies

Diet Group	Weight Loss (Kg)	P Value
Protein Content		
High (25%)	3.6	0.22
Low (15%)	3.0	
Fat Content		
High (40%)	3.3	0.94
Low (20%)	3.3	
Carbohydrate Content		
High (65%)	2.9	0.42
Low (35%)	3.4	

- All diets led to a modest reduction in average waist circumference, however there were no differences among the groups

- The low fat diets had slightly more favorable effects on LDL levels than the high fat diets

- The highest carbohydrate diet had slightly more favorable effects on LDL levels than the lowest carbohydrate diet, however the lowest carbohydrate diet had slightly more favorable effects on HDL levels

- Among all groups, blood pressure levels decreased by 1-2 mm Hg and the prevalence of the metabolic syndrome decreased, however there were no differences among the groups

- "Craving, fullness, and hunger and diet-satisfaction scores were similar at 6 months and at 2 years among the diets"

- Patients with higher attendance at dietary counseling sessions experienced more weight loss; attendance was similar among the four groups

Criticisms and Limitations: Compliance with each diet was imperfect, i.e. many patients did not consume the exact balance of nutrients that was recommended. However, since dietary compliance in "real-world" settings is imperfect, the results likely reflect "real-world" practice.

Patients in the study – all of whom volunteered to participate after receiving mass mailings – were highly motivated to lose weight. Outside of a research setting, patients might be less motivated, and therefore the benefits might not be as substantial.

Patients were offered regular weight loss counseling sessions throughout the two year study period. These services are not available in all health care settings.

Other Relevant Studies and Information:

- Some trials evaluating different dieting strategies have suggested that low-carbohydrate diets may lead to slightly greater weight loss than conventional low-fat diets in the short-term but not in the long-term (≥1 year of follow-up)[4,5,6,7,8,9]

- No high quality studies have compared the effects of different diets on "hard outcomes" such as cardiovascular disease or mortality

- Given the uncertainty about which dieting strategy is best, most guidelines suggest that patients choose whichever diet they are most likely to comply with while ensuring adequate intake of healthful foods containing necessary nutrients[10]

SUMMARY AND IMPLICATIONS:

Four diets with varying levels of fat, protein and carbohydrate content all resulted in modest weight loss over two years. There were no significant differences among the groups. Patients hoping to lose weight should select whichever diet program they are most likely to comply with while ensuring adequate intake of healthful foods containing necessary nutrients.

4 Shai et al. Weight loss with a low-carbohydrate, Mediterranean, or low-fat diet. N Engl J Med. 2008;359(3):229.

5 Gardner et al. Comparison of the Atkins, Zone, Ornish, and LEARN diets for change in weight and related risk factors among overweight premenopausal women: the A TO Z Weight Loss Study: a randomized trial. JAMA. 2007;297(9):969.

6 Samaha et al. A low-carbohydrate as compared with a low-fat diet in severe obesity. N Engl J Med. 2003;348(21):2074.

7 Foster et al. A randomized trial of a low-carbohydrate diet for obesity. N Engl J Med. 2003;348(21):2082.

8 Yancy et al. A low-carbohydrate, ketogenic diet vs. a low-fat diet to treat obesity and hyperlipidemia: a randomized, controlled trial. Ann Intern Med. 2004;140(10):769.

9 Nordmann et al. Effects of low-carbohydrate vs low-fat diets on weight loss and cardiovascular risk factors: a meta-analysis of randomized controlled trials. Arch Intern Med. 2006;166(3):285.

10 National Institutes of Health, National Heart, Lung, Blood Institute and the North American Association for the Study of Obesity. Practical guide identification, evaluation and treatment of overweight and obesity in adults, Publication no. 00-4084, Washington, DC 2000.

CLINICAL CASE: DIFFERENT DIETING STRATEGIES

CASE HISTORY:

A 40 year old man has struggled to lose weight for years. He has tried traditional low-fat diet many times, but always quickly regains the weight he loses. His BMI is 37.0, and he has hypertension and an elevated fasting blood glucose. He asks you whether he should try one of the new "fad diets" such as the "Atkins diet" or the "Zone diet" (both popular low carbohydrate diets).

Based on the results of this trial, what should you tell him?

SUGGESTED ANSWER:

The Atkins diet is an extremely low carbohydrate diet in which patients attempt to minimize the amount of carbohydrates they consume, while the Zone recommends a dietary composition of 40% carbohydrates, 30% protein, and 30% fat.

Existing evidence does not indicate that any one dieting strategy is superior to any other. In fact, one trial directly comparing the Atkins diet, the Zone diet, a low calorie "Weight Watchers" diet, and the "Ornish" low fat diet showed similar results with all four strategies[11].

Since this patient has not had success with traditional low fat dieting, it would be reasonable for him to experiment with alternative strategies. Whichever alternative he selects, he should make sure to consume sufficient quantities of healthful foods containing necessary nutrients. (Some experts worry that the Atkins diet does not provide adequate quantities of healthful foods, particularly in the early stages.) In addition, "fad diets" can be expensive, so you should warm this patient to be careful about costs.

Finally, since this patient has a BMI >35 with obesity-related complications (hypertension and impaired fasting glucose), he may be a candidate for bariatric surgery (see chapter on bariatric surgery).

---

11 Dansinger et al. Comparison of the Atkins, Ornish, Weight Watchers, and Zone diets for weight loss and heart disease risk reduction: a randomized trial. JAMA. 2005 Jan 5;293(1):43-53.

ASPIRIN FOR THE PRIMARY PREVENTION OF CARDIOVASCULAR DISEASE:

THE PHYSICIANS' HEALTH STUDY AND THE WOMEN'S HEALTH STUDY[12,13]

"[The Physicians' Health Study] demonstrates a conclusive reduction in the risk of myocardial infarction [in men], but the evidence concerning stroke and total cardiovascular deaths remains inconclusive ...as expected, [aspirin led to] increased risks of upper gastrointestinal ulcers and bleeding problems ..."

- The Physicians' Health Study Research Group[12]

---

12 The Physicians' Health Study Research Group. Final report on the aspirin component of the ongoing Physicians' Health Study. N Engl J Med. 1989 Jul 20;321(3):129-35.

13 Ridker et al. A randomized trial of low-dose aspirin in the primary prevention of cardiovascular disease in women. N Engl J Med. 2005 Mar 31;352(13):1293-304.

"[In the Women's Health Study] aspirin lowered the risk of stroke without affecting the risk of myocardial infarction or death from cardiovascular causes …as expected, the frequency of side effects related to bleeding and ulcers was increased …"

– Ridker et al.[13]

Research Question: Is aspirin effective for the prevention of cardiovascular disease in apparently healthy adults?

Funding: The Physicians' Health Study was sponsored by the National Institutes of Health and the Women's Health Study was sponsored by the National Heart, Lung, and Blood Institute and the National Cancer Institute.

Year Study Began: 1982 (Physicians' Health Study) and 1992 (Women's Health Study)

Year Study Published: 1989 (Physicians' Health Study) and 2005 (Women's Health Study)

Study Location: The Physicians' Health Study was open to apparently healthy male physicians throughout the U.S. who were mailed invitations to participate. The Women's Health Study was open to apparently healthy female health professionals throughout the U.S. who were mailed invitations to participate.

Who Was Studied: The Physicians' Health Study included apparently healthy male physician's 40-84 while the Women's Health Study included apparently healthy female health professionals ≥45.

Who Was Excluded: Patients were excluded from both trials if they had existing cardiovascular disease, cancer, other chronic medical problems, or if they were currently taking aspirin or non-steroidal anti-inflammatory agents. Both trials included a run-in period to identify patients unlikely to be compliant with the study protocol, and these patients were excluded before randomization.

How Many Patients: The Physicians' Health Study included 22,071 men while the Women's Health Study included 39,876 women.

Study Overview:

Figure 1: Summary of the Trials' Design

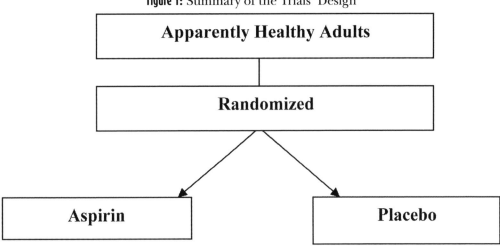

Study Intervention: In the Physicians' Health Study, patients in the aspirin group received aspirin 325 mg on alternate days while in the Women's Health Study patients in the aspirin group received aspirin 100 mg on alternate days. In both trials, patients in the control group received a placebo pill on alternate days.

Follow-Up: Approximately 5 years for the Physicians' Health Study and approximately 10 years for the Women's Health Study.

Endpoints: Myocardial infarction, stroke, cardiovascular mortality, and hemorrhagic side effects.

RESULTS:

Table 1: Summary of the Physicians' Health Study's Key Findings

Outcome	Aspirin Group	Placebo Group	P Value
Myocardial Infarction	1.3%	2.2%	<0.00001
Stroke	1.1%	0.9%	0.15
Cardiovascular Mortality	0.7%	0.8%	0.87
Gastrointestinal Ulcers	1.5%	1.3%	0.08
Bleeding Requiring Transfusion	0.4%	0.3%	0.02

Table 2: Summary of the Women's Health Study's Key Findings

Outcome	Aspirin Group	Placebo Group	P Value
Cardiovascular Events[a]	2.4%	2.6%	0.13
Stroke	1.1%	1.3%	0.04
Myocardial Infarction	1.0%	1.0%	0.83
Cardiovascular Mortality	0.6%	0.6%	0.68
Gastrointestinal Bleeding	4.6%	3.8%	<0.001

[a]Includes myocardial infarction, stroke, and death from cardiovascular causes.

- in both trial's, aspirin was most beneficial among older patients (men ≥50 and women ≥65)

Criticisms and Limitations: In the Physicians' Health Study, aspirin 325 mg was given on alternate days while in the Women's Health Study aspirin 100 mg was given on alternate days. In clinical practice, however, most patients receive aspirin 81 mg daily (data concerning the optimal ASA dose are sparse).

Both of these trials are limited in generalizability. Both included patients of high socioeconomic status. In addition, patients found to be non-compliant during a run-in period were excluded. Patients in the general population are likely to be less compliant with therapy, and therefore the benefits of aspirin observed in "real-world" settings may be lower.

Other Relevant Studies and Information:

- Other trials of aspirin for cardiovascular disease prevention have also suggested that aspirin reduces the risk of cardiovascular events while increasing bleeding risk[14].

- Whether aspirin has a differential effect on men and women is unclear: one meta-analysis suggested that in men aspirin may preferentially prevent myocardial infarctions while in women aspirin may preferentially

---

14 Antithrombotic Trialists' (ATT) Collaboration. Aspirin in the primary and secondary prevention of vascular disease: collaborative meta-analysis of individual participant data from randomised trials. Lancet. 2009;373(9678):1849.

prevent strokes[15]. Other experts believe this conclusion is premature, however[16].

- Aspirin is also effective in preventing cardiovascular events in high risk patients with vascular disease[17], and the absolute benefits are greater among these patients.

The American Heart Association recommends daily aspirin for apparently healthy men and women whose 10 year risk of a first event exceeds 10% while the United States Preventive Services Task Force recommends low-dose (e.g. 75 mg) daily aspirin for primary cardiovascular prevention in the following circumstances:

- in women 55-79 when the reduction in ischemic stroke risk is greater than the increase in gastrointestinal hemorrhage risk (e.g. a woman with a high stroke risk but low bleeding risk would be a good candidate while a woman with a high bleeding risk but low stroke risk would not be)

- in men 45-79 when the reduction in the risk of myocardial infarction is greater than the increase in gastrointestinal hemorrhage risk (e.g. a man with a high risk of myocardial infarction but low bleeding risk would be a good candidate while a man with a high bleeding risk but low risk of myocardial infarction would not be)

SUMMARY AND IMPLICATIONS:

In apparently healthy men and women, aspirin leads to a small reduction in the risk of cardiovascular disease while increasing bleeding risk. In men, aspirin may preferentially prevent myocardial infarctions, while in women aspirin may preferentially prevent strokes, though this conclusion is uncertain. Aspirin is recommended for primary cardiovascular prevention in both men and women with cardiovascular risk factors when the risk of gastrointestinal hemorrhage is low.

---

15 Berger et al. Aspirin for the primary prevention of cardiovascular events in women and men: a sex-specific meta-analysis of randomized controlled trials. JAMA. 2006;295(3):306.

16 Hennekens et al. Sex-related differences in response to aspirin in cardiovascular disease: an untested hypothesis. Nature Clinical Practice Cardiovascular Medicine. (2006) 3, 4-5.

17 Berger et al. Low-dose aspirin in patients with stable cardiovascular disease: a meta-analysis. Am J Med. 2008;121(1):43.

CLINICAL CASE: ASPIRIN FOR THE PRIMARY PREVENTION OF CARDIOVASCULAR DISEASE

CASE HISTORY:

A 60 year old woman with a history of hypertension, hyperlipidemia, liver cirrhosis, esophageal varices, and recurrent gastrointestinal bleeding asks whether she should receive aspirin to reduce her risk of cardiovascular disease. Based on the results of the Women's Health Study, what would you recommend?

SUGGESTED ANSWER:

The Women's Health Study demonstrated that, in female health professionals ≥45, daily aspirin leads to a small but detectable reduction in the risk of cardiovascular disease while increasing bleeding risk. The United States Preventive Services Task Force recommends low-dose daily aspirin in women 55-79 when the reduction in cardiovascular risk is judged to be greater than the increase in risk of gastrointestinal hemorrhage.

The patient in this vignette has risk factors for cardiovascular disease and therefore would ordinarily be a good candidate for aspirin. However, she also has numerous risk factors for gastrointestinal bleeding, making aspirin therapy risky. Overall, the risks of aspirin likely outweigh the benefits in this patient.

POSTMENOPAUSAL HORMONE THERAPY:

THE WOMEN'S HEALTH INITIATIVE (WHI) [18]

"The [Women's Health Initiative] provides an important health answer for generations of healthy postmenopausal women to come—do not use estrogen/progestin to prevent chronic disease."

- Fletcher and Colditz [19]

Research Question: Should postmenopausal women take combined hormone therapy for the prevention of cardiovascular disease and fractures?

---

18 The Women's Health Initiative Investigators. Risks and benefits of estrogen plus progestin in healthy postmenopausal women: principal results from the Women's Health Initiative randomized controlled trial. JAMA. 2002 Jul 17;288(3):321-33.

19 Fletcher SW, Colditz GA. Failure of estrogen plus progestin therapy for prevention. JAMA. 2002;288:366-368.

Funding: The National Heart, Lung, and Blood Institute.

Year Study Began: 1993

Year Study Published: 2002

Study Location: 40 clinical centers throughout the U.S.

Who Was Studied: Postmenopausal women 50-79 years of age.

Who Was Excluded: Patients with a prior hysterectomy, those with another serious medical condition associated with a life expectancy of less than three years, or those with a history of cancer.

How Many Patients: 16,608

Study Overview:

Figure 1: Summary of the WHI's Design

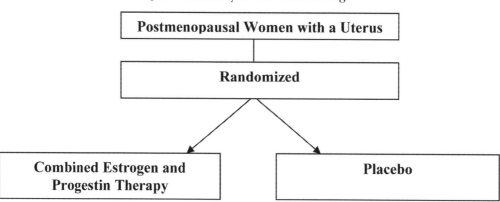

Study Intervention: Patients in the combined hormone therapy group received one tablet of conjugated equine estrogen 0.625 mg and medroxyprogesterone acetate 2.5 mg daily. Patients in the control group received a placebo tablet.

Follow-Up: Mean of 5.6 years[20] (8.5 years of therapy were planned, but the intervention was stopped early because initial results showed that the health risks exceeded the benefits)

Endpoints: Primary outcomes: coronary heart disease (nonfatal or fatal myocardial infarction) and invasive breast cancer. Other major outcomes: stroke,

---

20 The follow-up was originally reported as 5.2 years but more accurately was 5.6 years according to Dr. Rowan Chlebowski, a member of the Women's Health Initiative's Steering Committee.

pulmonary embolism, hip fracture, death, and a global index summarizing the risks and benefits of combined hormone therapy.

RESULTS:

- the global index score summarizing the risks and benefits of combined hormone therapy suggested a small overall harm from combined hormone therapy

Table 1: The WHI's Key Findings

Outcome	Combined Hormone Therapy Group[a]	Placebo Group[a]	Statistically Significant?[b]
Myocardial infarctions	0.37%	0.30%	borderline
Stroke	0.29%	0.21%	yes
Venous thromboembolic disease	0.34%	0.16%	yes
Invasive breast cancer	0.38%	0.30%	borderline
Hip fracture	0.10%	0.15%	yes
Mortality	0.52%	0.53%	no

[a]Percentages represent average annualized rates, i.e. the percentage of people who experienced each outcome per year.
[b]Exact P values not reported.

Criticisms and Limitations: The trial only tested one dose and one formulation of combined hormone therapy. It is possible that the risks and benefits are different when lower doses or different formulations of estrogens and progestins are used.

Other Relevant Studies and Information:

- Observational studies (case control and cohort studies) prior to the WHI suggested that combined hormone therapy decreased the risk of cardiovascular disease[21,22]. It is now believed that these studies came to erroneous conclusions because women taking combined hormone therapy tended to be healthier than those who weren't, making it appear as though combined hormone therapy reduced the risk of cardiovascular disease.

- The HERS trial showed that, among women with existing heart disease, there was a higher rate of venous thromboembolism among women who took combined hormone therapy[23].

- The WHI included a separate evaluation of unopposed estrogen therapy (without a progestin) in women with prior hysterectomies. This study suggested an increased rate of stroke among users of estrogen therapy, but the rates of heart attacks and breast cancer were similar in the estrogen and placebo groups[24].

- An 11-year follow-up evaluation of patients in the WHI showed that breast cancers among women who took combined hormone therapy were more likely to be advanced stage, and that breast cancer mortality rates were higher compared to women in the placebo group[25].

SUMMARY AND IMPLICATIONS:

The WHI showed that the risks (cardiovascular disease and breast cancer) of combined hormone therapy outweigh the benefits (a reduction in fractures). Since the absolute risks are small, combined hormone therapy remains an option for the management of postmenopausal symptoms, however combined hormone therapy should only be used when other therapies have failed. The WHI also contains an important lesson for the medical community: except in unusual circumstances, randomized trials – not case-control or cohort studies – are needed before new therapies become the standard of care.

21 Stampfer M, Colditz G. Estrogen replacement therapy and coronary heart disease: a quantitative assessment of the epidemiologic evidence. *Prev Med.* 1991;20:47-63.

22 Grady D, Rueben SB, Pettiti DB, et al. Combined hormone therapy to prevent disease and prolong life in postmenopausal women. *Ann Intern Med.* 1992;117:1016-1037.

23 Hulley et al. Noncardiovascular disease outcomes during 6.8 years of combined hormone therapy: Heart and Estrogen/progestin Replacement Study follow-up (HERS II). JAMA 2002 Jul 3;288(1):58-66.

24 Anderson et al. Effects of conjugated equine estrogen in postmenopausal women with hysterectomy: the Women's Health Initiative randomized controlled trial. JAMA 2004 Apr 14;291(14):1701-12.

25 Chlebowski et al. Estrogen plus progestin and breast cancer incidence and mortality in postmenopausal women. *JAMA.* 2010;304(15):1684-1692.

CLINICAL CASE: POSTMENOPAUSAL HORMONE THERAPY

CASE HISTORY:

A 52 year old woman with an intact uterus reports persistent and bothersome hot flashes and vaginal dryness since undergoing menopause one year ago. The symptoms have not responded to relaxation techniques, and she asks about the possibility of starting hormone therapy to control the symptoms.

Based on the results of the Women's Health Initiative, what can you tell her about the risks of hormone therapy?

SUGGESTED ANSWER:

The Women's Health Initiative suggested that long term (>5 years) combined estrogen and progestin therapy is associated with increased rates of myocardial infarction, stroke, venous thromboembolism, and breast cancer, and a reduced rate of hip fractures. However, given that the absolute increase in disease rates is small, short term (ideally two to three years) hormone therapy is an acceptable treatment for bothersome menopausal symptoms that do not respond to other therapies.

Women in the Women's Health Initiative received hormone therapy for a mean of 5.6 years; the risks of short term therapy are likely to be lower. In addition, women in the study received conjugated equine estrogen 0.625 mg and medroxyprogesterone acetate 2.5 mg daily. Some experts believe that hormone preparations with lower doses may be safer although there are no data to support these claims.

THE EUROPEAN RANDOMIZED STUDY OF SCREENING FOR PROSTATE CANCER (ERSPC)[26,27]

"[The ERSPC showed] a relative reduction of 21% in the rate of death from prostate cancer in the screening group ... [but this] reduction was achieved after considerable use of resources ... [and there was no] significant between-group difference in all-cause mortality."

- Dr. Anthony B. Miller[28]

---

26 Schröder et al. Screening and prostate-cancer mortality in a randomized European study. N Engl J Med. 2009 Mar 26;360(13):1320-8.

27 Schröder et al. Prostate-cancer mortality at 11 years of follow-up. N Engl J Med. 2012 Mar 15;366(11):981-90.

28 Miller AB. New data on prostate-cancer mortality after PSA screening. N Engl J Med. 2012 Mar 15;366(11):1047-48.

Research Question: Is screening for prostate cancer with prostate-specific-antigen (PSA) testing effective?

Funding: Europe Against Cancer, the European Union, local grants, and an unrestricted grant from Beckman Coulter, which manufactures PSA tests.

Year Study Began: 1991

Year Study Published: 2012

Study Location: Numerous sites in 7 European countries (The Netherlands, Belgium, Sweden, Finland, Italy, Spain, and Switzerland)

Who Was Studied: Men between the ages of 55 and 69.

How Many Patients: 162,388

Study Overview:

Figure 1: Summary of the Trial's Design

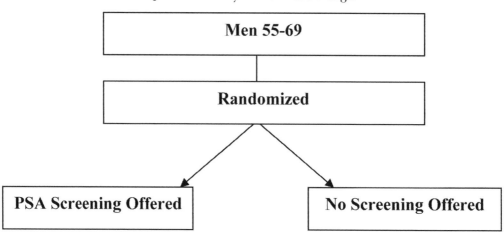

Study Intervention: The study protocols varied slightly from country to country. In the screening group, men were typically offered screening every 4 years, and most were only screened with a PSA test (though some men also received a digital rectal examination and/or transrectal ultrasound). Men with a PSA ≥3.0 ng/ml were typically referred for prostate biopsy, however in some countries a higher cutoff (typically 4.0 ng/ml) was used. Most men who underwent biopsies received sextant (6-core) biopsies guided by transrectal ultrasonography. Men with positive biopsies were treated at the discretion of their physicians, i.e. no standard treatment protocols were specified.

In the control group, men were not invited for PSA screening as part of the trial, though a small percentage may have received PSA screening outside of the study protocol.

Follow-Up: Median of 11 years

Endpoints: Primary outcome: Death from prostate cancer. Secondary outcomes: Prostate cancer diagnoses, all-cause mortality.

RESULTS:

- 82.2% of men in the screening group were screened at least once (i.e. 17.8% declined screening), and those who were screened received an average of 2.3 screenings

- 16.6% of screening tests were positive (i.e. PSA ≥3.0)

- 85.9% of men who had a positive screening test agreed to undergo biopsy, and 24.1% of men who underwent a biopsy were found to have cancer

- In total, 9.6% of men in the screening group were diagnosed with prostate cancer vs. 6.0% of men in the control group

- prostate cancers detected in the screening group were less advanced (lower stage and Gleason score) than those detected in the control group

Table 1: Summary of the Trial's Key Findings[a]

Outcome	Screening Group	Control Group	P Value
Prostate Cancer Mortality	0.39	0.50	0.001
All-Cause Mortality	18.2	18.5	0.50

[a]Event rates are per 1000 person-years, i.e. the number of deaths that occurred for every 1000 years of participant time. For example, 0.39 deaths per 1000 person-years means that, on average, there were 0.39 deaths among 100 subjects who were each enrolled in the trial for ten years.

- the authors calculated that 936 men would need to be offered screening and 33 additional men would need to be diagnosed with prostate cancer to prevent one death from prostate cancer (including all available follow-up data for ≥12 years)

Criticisms and Limitations: It is likely that some men (approximately 20%) in the control group received prostate cancer screening from their physicians outside of the study protocol (referred to as "contamination"). The authors did not estimate the rate at which contamination occurred, however if it occurred frequently it would have lead to an underestimation of both the benefits and harms of screening.

This was a preliminary report from the ERSPC trial, which is ongoing. Future analyses will provide long term follow-up data, as well as quality of life analyses. It is possible that the impact of screening may be more favorable with longer follow-up.

Men in this study were generally screened every four years, however in many countries (including the U.S.) men are screened more frequently (e.g. every 1-2 years). More frequent screening would presumably improve the benefits of screening, but would also increase harms from false positive results (i.e. over-diagnosis and overtreatment of early-stage cancers that would never cause harm in the patient's lifetime).

Most men with positive screening tests in the study underwent sextant (6-core) biopsies, however many urologists now recommend extended core biopsies in which a larger portion of the prostate is sampled. While extended core biopsies increase the sensitivity for prostate cancer, they are also associated with more false positive results.

The study was not adequately powered to detect small reductions in all-cause mortality between the screening and control groups.

Other Relevant Studies and Information:

- 14 year follow-up data were reported from one of the sites where this trial took place. Data from this site, where patients were screened every two years, showed a more substantial reduction in prostate cancer death (just 293 men needed to be screened and 12 diagnosed with prostate cancer to prevent one prostate cancer death). There was no reduction in all-cause mortality, however[29].

- Another large randomized trial in the U.S. did not show a benefit of prostate cancer screening with annual PSA measurements and digital rectal examination, however some patients in the control group received

---

29 Hugosson et al. Mortality results from the Göteborg randomised population-based prostate-cancer screening trial. Lancet Oncol. 2010 Aug;11(8):725-32.

screening from their physicians outside of the study protocol, which may have affected the results[30,31].

- Early stage prostate cancer is commonly treated with surgery or radiation therapy (though a strategy of close monitoring with "active surveillance" is also a recommended approach). Complications of surgery and radiation include urinary incontinence, sexual dysfunction, and bowel problems. Since prostate cancer screening leads to an increase in the diagnosis of prostate cancer, screening will likely lead to an increase in the rates of these complications.

- In 2011, the United States Preventive Services Task Force drafted new guidelines recommending against routine prostate cancer screening because the potential harms from screening (unnecessary surgeries and radiation therapy) may not outweigh the small benefits[32].

SUMMARY AND IMPLICATIONS:

Screening for prostate cancer with PSA testing every four years leads to a small but significant reduction in prostate cancer deaths along with a substantial increase in the (potentially unnecessary) diagnosis and treatment of prostate cancer. There was no effect of screening on all-cause mortality, though the study was not powered for this analysis. The ERSPC trial is ongoing, and future analyses will provide longer term follow-up data. In the meantime, draft guidelines from the United States Preventive Services Task Force recommend against routine screening.

CLINICAL CASE: SCREENING FOR PROSTATE CANCER

CASE HISTORY:

A 50 year-old African American man whose father died from prostate cancer at the age of 64 presents to your clinic for a routine evaluation. Based on

---

30 Andriole et al. Mortality results from a randomized prostate-cancer screening trial. N Engl J Med 2009;360:1310-1319.

31 Andriole et al. Prostate cancer screening in the randomized Prostate, Lung, Colorectal, and Ovarian Cancer Screening Trial: mortality results after 13 years of follow-up. J Natl Cancer Inst 2012;104:1-8.

32 Chou et al. Screening for Prostate Cancer: A Review of the Evidence for the U.S. Preventive Services Task Force. Ann Intern Med. 2011 Dec 6;155(11):762-71.

the results of the ERSPC trial, do you recommend prostate cancer screening for this patient?

SUGGESTED ANSWER:

The ERSPC trial found that screening for prostate cancer with PSA testing every four years leads to a small reduction in prostate cancer deaths along with a substantial increase in the (potentially unnecessary) diagnosis and treatment of prostate cancer. There was no effect of screening on all-cause mortality, though the study was not powered for this analysis. Based on the results of ERSPC and a large U.S. prostate cancer screening trial, draft guidelines from the United States Preventive Services Task Force recommend against routine screening.

However, the patient in this vignette is at particularly high risk for developing prostate cancer (African American men, as well as men with a family history of prostate cancer, are at increased risk). For this reason, some experts might advocate screening for this patient.

On the other hand, there is no evidence to suggest that PSA screening is any more effective for identifying dangerous cancers among high risk patients. In fact, since PSA levels tend to be higher among African American men than among white men, it is possible that the man in this vignette would be at particularly high risk for being inappropriately diagnosed with a slow-growing prostate cancer that would never impact his life. (The percentage of patients in ERSPC who were African American or who had a family history of prostate cancer was not specified.)

Thus, there is no correct answer to the question of whether or not this patient should be screened. You might inform this man that prostate cancer screening is no longer recommended for most men, however it would be reasonable to consider screening in his case because he is at increased risk. Should he express an interest in screening, you should inform him of the associated risks (the potentially unnecessary diagnosis and treatment of a slow-growing cancer that otherwise would not impact his life) before proceeding.

THE COCHRANE REVIEW OF SCREENING MAMMOGRAPHY[33]

"For every 2000 women invited for screening throughout 10 years, one will have her life prolonged ... [and] 10 healthy women who would not have had a breast cancer diagnosis if there had not been screening will be diagnosed as cancer patients, and will be treated unnecessarily ..."

- Gøtzsche and Nielsen[33]

Research Question: Is screening mammography effective?

Funding: The Cochrane Collaboration, an independent, non-profit organization supported by governments, universities, hospital trusts, charities and donations. The Cochrane Collaboration does not accept commercial funding.

Year Study Began: The earliest trial began in 1963 and the most recent began in 1991.

---

33 Gøtzsche PC and Nielsen M. Screening for breast cancer with mammography. Cochrane Database Syst Rev. 2011 Jan 19;(1):CD001877.

Year Study Published: The results of the individual trials were published during the 1970's, 1980's, 1990's, and 2000's. This Cochrane review was published in 2011.

Study Location: The trials were conducted in Sweden, the U.S., Canada, and the United Kingdom.

Study Overview: This was a meta-analysis of randomized clinical trials of screening mammography in women without previously diagnosed breast cancer.

Which Trials Were Included.

A total of 11 randomized trials were identified using an exhaustive search strategy, however three were not eligible for inclusion because of methodological limitations and one was excluded due to bias. Therefore, 7 trials were included in the meta-analysis. These trials are listed below with the country and start date in parentheses:

- The Health Insurance Plan trial (USA 1963)

- The Malmö trial (Sweden 1978)

- The Two-County trial (Sweden 1977)

- The Canadian trials (two trials with different age groups) (Canada 1980)

- The Stockholm trial (Sweden 1981)

- The Göteborg trial (Sweden 1982)

- The United Kingdom age trial (United Kingdom 1991)

Study Intervention:

In all 7 trials, women were randomized to receive either an invitation for breast cancer screening with mammography or no invitation for screening. Women in the screening group were invited for 2-9 rounds of screening, depending on the trial.

RESULTS:

- data were available for 599,090 women over 13 years of follow-up

- the authors judged 3 of the 7 trials to have optimal randomization methodology; for these 3 trials, data were available for 292,153 women

Table 1: Summary of Key Findings, 13 Years of Follow-Up

Outcome	Relative Risk with Screening (95% Confidence Intervals)
Breast Cancer Mortality	
All 7 trials	0.81 (0.74-0.87)
3 trials with optimal methodology	0.90 (0.79-1.02)
All-Cause Mortality	
All 7 trials	Unreliable[a]
3 trials with optimal methodology	0.99 (0.95-1.03)
Surgeries[b]	
All 7 trials	1.35 (1.26-1.44)
3 trials with optimal methodology	1.31 (1.22-1.44)
Radiotherapy	
All 7 trials	1.32 (1.16-1.50)
3 trials with optimal methodology	1.24 (1.04-1.49)

[a]The authors felt this number was unreliable, and therefore do not report it.
[b]Mastectomies and lumpectomies

Criticisms and Limitations: Many of the individual trials included in this meta-analysis suffered from methodological flaws. Some of these flaws may have biased the results in favor of the screening group while others may have biased the results in favor of the controls:

- In many cases women assigned to the control groups appeared to be systematically different from those assigned to the screening groups. For example, in the Two-County trial more women in the control group than in the screening group had been diagnosed with breast cancer prior to the start of the trial. Differences such as these may have biased the results.

- Determination of breast cancer mortality rates in many of the trials was potentially biased or inaccurate. The physicians who determined the cause of death for study subjects were frequently aware of whether the subjects had been assigned to the screening vs. control groups, and it is possible that their judgments were influenced by this knowledge. Furthermore, few autopsies of patients who died were performed, and therefore many of the cause-of-death determinations may have been inaccurate.

- Some experts have criticized the screening mammography trials because, particularly in some of the trials, women in the control groups began receiving screening before the trials were concluded. Because it presumably takes several years before the benefits of screening are apparent, it is unlikely this would have substantially affected the trial results. Still, it is possible that mammograms among controls partially obscured the benefits of screening.

- Some women in these trials received 1-view mammograms rather than the standard 2-view studies. It is possible that the 1-view films were less effective at identifying cancers.

- These trials were all conducted several years ago. Breast cancer treatments have improved in recent years, and some experts believe that with current treatment options, the benefits of early detection of breast cancer may be smaller[34].

Other Relevant Studies and Information:

- A recent modeling study suggests that screening mammography every two years "achieves most of the benefit of annual screening with less harm." In addition, this study suggests that screening mammograms in women between the ages of 40 to 49 lead to only a small benefit but a high rate of false positive results[35].

- Table 2 lists breast cancer screening guidelines from two organizations

---

34 Welch HG. Screening mammography – a long run for a short slide? N Engl J Med. 2010 Sep 23;363(13):1276-8.

35 Mandelblatt et al. Effects of mammography screening under different screening schedules: model estimates of potential benefits and harms. Ann Intern Med. 2009;151:738-47.

Table 2: Major Breast Cancer Screening Guidelines

Guideline	Recommendations
The United States Preventive Services Task Force	• screening recommended every 2 years for women 50-74 years of age • "the decision to start [screening] before the age of 50 years should be an individual one and take patient context into account …"
The American Cancer Society	• yearly mammograms are recommended starting at age 40 and continuing for as long as a woman is in good health

SUMMARY AND IMPLICATIONS:

Most of the trials of screening mammography have considerable methodological flaws. Despite these limitations, the Cochrane Review suggests that screening mammography modestly reduces breast cancer mortality but may not reduce all-cause mortality. In addition, screening mammography leads to the diagnosis and unnecessary treatment of a substantial number of women who may never have developed symptoms of breast cancer. According to the authors, for every 2000 women offered screening mammograms over a 10-year period, 1 will have her life prolonged while 10 will be treated for breast cancer unnecessarily. The optimal use of screening mammography remains an area of considerable controversy.

CLINICAL CASE: SCREENING MAMMOGRAPHY

CASE HISTORY:

A 68 year old woman with chronic obstructive pulmonary disease, diabetes, and osteoporosis visits your clinic for a routine visit. When you mention that she is due for a screening mammogram, she protests: "I have so many other medical problems. Why do we need to look for more?"

Based on the results of the Cochrane Review on mammography, what can you tell this patient about the risks and benefits of screening mammography?

SUGGESTED ANSWER:

The Cochrane Mammography review suggests that screening mammography modestly reduces breast cancer mortality but may not reduce all-cause mortality. In addition, screening mammography leads to the diagnosis and unnecessary treatment of a substantial number of women who may never have developed symptoms of breast cancer. Some women may not feel that this trade-off is worth it.

The woman in this vignette has other significant co-morbidities, and does not want to "look for more." Thus, it would be perfectly reasonable for her to opt not to undergo screening. Since this patient is in poor health, screening may not even be appropriate for her since the benefits of screening occur several years down the road and she may not live long enough to realize these benefits. Indeed, the American Cancer Society only recommends screening among women in good overall health.

THE HUMAN PAPILLOMAVIRUS VACCINE:

THE FUTURE II TRIAL[36]

"In the Future II trial, [3.6% of] vaccinated women received [a diagnosis of grade 2 or 3 cervical intraepithelial neoplasia or adenocarcinoma in situ] over an average of 3 years, as compared with [4.4% of] unvaccinated women ... [Still] a cautious approach may be warranted in light of important unanswered questions about overall vaccine effectiveness, duration of protection, and adverse effects that may emerge over time."

- Sawaya and Smith-McCune[37]

Research Question: Is the quadrivalent human papillomavirus (HPV) vaccine against HPV types 6, 11, 16, and 18 safe and effective?

36 The Future II Study Group. Quadrivalent vaccine against human papillomavirus to prevent high-grade cervical lesions. NEJM. 2007;356:1915-1927.

37 Sawaya GF and Smith-McCune K. HPV Vaccination – More answers, more questions. NEJM 2007;356:1991-93.

- HPV-16 and HPV-18 cause 70% of all cervical cancers

- HPV-6 and HPV-11 cause the majority of anogenital warts

Funding: Merck

Year Study Began: 2002

Year Study Published: 2007

Study Location: 90 study sites in 13 countries in both the developed and developing world

Who Was Studied: Girls and women 15 – 26 years old

Who Was Excluded: Women who were pregnant, those who reported abnormal Papanicolaou (Pap) smear results at baseline, and those with >4 sexual partners.

How Many Patients: 12,167

Study Overview:

Figure 1: **Summary of FUTURE II's Design**

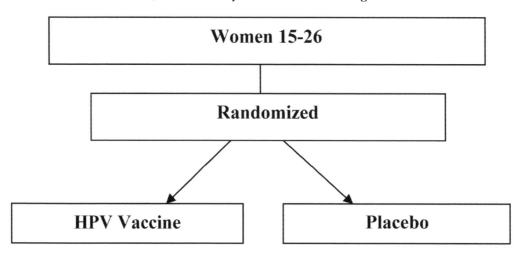

Study Intervention: Women assigned to the HPV vaccine group received the vaccine upon enrollment, at two months, and at six months. Women assigned to the placebo group received a placebo injection according to the same schedule.

Women in both groups underwent Pap smears and anogenital swabs for HPV DNA testing at baseline and at 1, 6, 24, 36, and 48 months after the third vaccine (or placebo) injection.

Patients with abnormal Pap smears were managed according to standard protocols.

Follow-Up: A mean of 3 years

Endpoints: Primary outcome: A composite of high-grade cervical lesions due to HPV-16 and HPV-18 including cervical intraepithelial neoplasia (CIN) grades 2 or 3, adenocarcinoma in situ, or invasive cervical cancer. Secondary outcome: High-grade cervical lesions due to any HPV type.

- CIN is a precancerous dysplastic lesion that is a precursor to squamous cell carcinoma of the cervix (the most common type of cervical cancer in the U.S.)

- CIN is graded on a scale of 1-3; CIN 1 is a low-grade lesion that frequently regresses and is managed with close monitoring; CIN 2 and CIN 3 are high grade lesions that, if left untreated, often progress to invasive cancer

- Adenocarcinoma in situ is another type of precancerous dysplastic lesion that may progress to adenocarcinoma (adenocarcinoma represents about 25% of cervical cancers in the U.S.)

RESULTS:

- There were no cases of invasive cervical cancer during the study period in either group

- Vaccine side effects appeared to be minor, though patients in the vaccine group did report slightly higher rates of injection site pain, seasonal allergies, and neck pain than patients in the placebo group

Table 1: Summary of Future II's Key Findings[a]

Outcome	HPV Vaccine Group	Placebo Group	P Value[b]
High grade lesions due to HPV-16 or HPV-18[c]	<0.1	0.3	Significant
High grade lesions due to any HPV type[d]	1.3	1.5	Significant

[a]Rates are per 100 person-years, i.e. the number of events that occurred for every 100 years of participant time. For example, 0.3 events per 100 person-years means that there were, on average, 0.3 events among 50 subjects who were each enrolled in the trial for two years.
[b]Actual p values not reported.
[c]Only includes patients who were negative for HPV-16 and HPV-18 at baseline and the one month post-vaccination visit, and who closely followed the study protocol.
[d]Includes all enrolled patients, including those who had HPV-16 or HPV-18 at baseline and those who did not follow the study protocol closely. This analysis may better mimic "real-world" clinical practice.

- HPV vaccination did not appear to prevent the development of high-grade cervical lesions due to HPV-16 or HPV-18 among patients already infected with these HPV types at baseline

- 99% of women who received the vaccine developed detectable levels of neutralizing HPV antibodies after vaccination, however only 68% continued to have detectable antibody levels against the HPV-18 serotype at month 24

Criticisms and Limitations: Although HPV vaccination led to a significant reduction in the rates of high-grade cervical lesions, the absolute reduction was modest ("129 women would need to be vaccinated in order to prevent one case of grade 2 or 3 cervical intraepithelial, neoplasia or adenocarcinoma in situ" during three years of follow-up[37]). Some experts have argued that this relatively small benefit does not justify HPV vaccination given the uncertainty about long term vaccine safety and effectiveness.

HPV vaccination led to a reduction in precancerous cervical lesions but not a reduction in cervical cancer (cervical cancer rates are extremely low with effective cervical cancer screening). Because many precancerous lesions do not progress to cervical cancer, particularly with effective cervical cancer screening, the reduction in cancer rates from HPV vaccination is likely to be considerably smaller than the reduction in rates of precancerous lesions observed in this trial.

Although the effectiveness of HPV vaccination did not appear to wane during the course of the study, only 68% of patients continued to have detectable antibody levels for the HPV-18 serotype at month 24. Follow-up data from Future II will be needed to determine whether the effectiveness of HPV vaccination persists beyond three years of follow-up.

Other Relevant Studies and Information:

- The Future I trial, which included fewer patients than Future II, showed that HPV vaccination led to a modest absolute reduction in composite rates of CIN 1, 2, and 3, and a modest absolute reduction in the rates of anogenital and vaginal warts[38]

- The Patricia trial showed that a bivalent HPV vaccine against HPV-16 and HPV-18 was modestly effective in preventing CIN 2

- Another trial showed that the quadrivalent HPV vaccine reduces the rates of HPV infection and the "development of related external genital lesions in males 16 to 26 years of age"[39], as well as the rates of anal intraepithelial neoplasia (a precursor to anal cancer)[40]

- Both the quadrivalent and bivalent HPV vaccines have been approved in the U.S. and are recommended for girls 11-12 years of age and for girls and women ≤26 who did not receive the vaccine when they were younger; the quadrivalent vaccine has also been approved for use in males 9-26

SUMMARY AND IMPLICATIONS:

The quadrivalent HPV vaccine led to a modest absolute reduction in high-grade cervical lesions that are precursors to cervical cancer in girls and women 15 - 26. The vaccine is now recommended for girls 11-12 years of age and for girls and women ≤26 who did not receive the vaccine when they were younger. Some experts remain cautious, however, because the absolute benefits of the vaccine are small and of uncertain duration, and may not justify yet unknown safety risks.

---

38 Garland et al. Quadrivalent vaccine against human papillomavirus to prevent anogenital disease. NEJM. 2007;356:1928.

39 Giuliano et al. Efficacy of quadrivalent HPV vaccine against HPV Infection and disease in males. N Engl J Med. 2011;364(5):401.

40 Palefsky et al. HPV vaccine against anal HPV infection and anal intraepithelial neoplasia. N Engl J Med. 2011 Oct 27;365(17):1576-85.

CLINICAL CASE: HUMAN PAPILLOMAVIRUS VACCINATION

CASE HISTORY:

You are evaluating a 12 year-old girl during her routine annual check-up. When you mention to her that the Centers for Disease Control recommend HPV vaccination for 11 and 12 year old girls, she appears apprehensive. She says, "I hate shots. Do I really need this vaccine?" Upon further questioning, the girl also tells you that she is not currently sexually active and does not plan on becoming sexually active in the near future.

What can you tell this girl about the risks and benefits of HPV vaccination based on the results of Future II?

SUGGESTED ANSWER:

Future II demonstrated the effectiveness of the quadrivalent HPV vaccine in preventing high grade cervical lesions that are precursors of cervical cancer. Girls and women are probably most likely to benefit from vaccination prior to the onset of sexual activity when they are at risk for acquiring HPV infections. As this girl's doctor, you might emphasize that although she is not planning on becoming sexually active in the near future, it is best for her to receive the vaccine before she does become sexually active.

On the other hand, the absolute benefits of the vaccine are relatively modest. In addition, we do not yet know whether there are any long term safety concerns with the vaccine, or even if the vaccine will remain effective in preventing HPV infection in the long term.

You might handle this situation by recommending the vaccine to your patient (and her family), but inform her that it would also be reasonable to decline. Regardless of whether or not she decides to be vaccinated, your patient should receive regular Pap smears when she reaches the appropriate age (21 according to guidelines from the American College of Obstetrics and Gynecology).

SECTION 2:

INTERNAL MEDICINE

ARRHYTHMIA SUPPRESSION FOLLOWING MYOCARDIAL INFARCTION:

THE CAST TRIAL[41,42]

"The CAST study has demonstrated that the use of [the antiarrhythmic medications encainide and flecainide] . . . after myocardial infarction carries a risk of excess mortality."

- Echt et al.[41]

Research Question: Do anti-arrhythmic medications – which were widely used to suppress ventricular arrhythmias prior to the publication of CAST – improve survival in patients with recent myocardial infarctions?

Funding: National Heart, Lung, and Blood Institute.

41 Echt et al. Mortality and morbidity in patients receiving encainide, flecainide, or placebo. N Engl J Med. 1991 Mar 21;324(12):781-788.

42 The Cardiac Arrhythmia Suppression Trial II Investigators. Effect of the antiarrhythmic agent moricizine on survival after myocardial infarction. N Engl J Med. 1992 Jul 23;327:227-233.

Year Study Began: 1987

Year Study Published: 1991

Study Location: Multiple centers throughout the U.S.

Who Was Studied: Patients who had suffered a recent (within the past six days to 2 years) myocardial infarction and who had an average of ≥6 ventricular premature depolarizations per hour on ambulatory electrocardiographic monitoring. In addition, patients were required to have a depressed ejection fraction.

Who Was Excluded: Patients with extended runs of ventricular tachycardia. In addition, prior to the start of the trial, patients were enrolled in a pilot study in which they were given the study medications, and those with a poor response (i.e. those whose arrhythmias were not effectively suppressed) were excluded.

How Many Patients: 2,653

Study Overview:

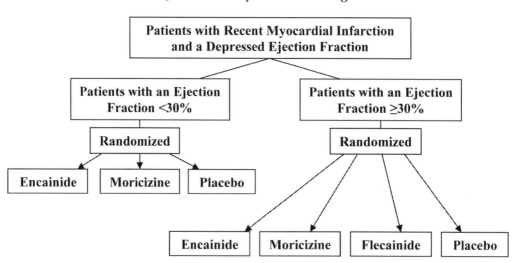

Figure 1: Summary of CAST's Design

Study Intervention: Patients with an ejection fraction under 30% were randomly assigned to receive either encainide, moricizine, or a placebo (these patients were not given flecainide to "avoid potential aggravation of left ventricular dysfunction"). Patients with an ejection fraction of at least 30% were randomized to any of the three study medications (encainide, flecainide, or moricizine) or to placebo.

Follow-Up: Mean of 10 months for the encainide and flecainide arms and 18 months for the morcizine arm.

Endpoints: Primary outcome: an arrhythmia leading to death or cardiac arrest. Secondary outcome: death or cardiac arrest due to all causes.

RESULTS:

- the trial arms involving encainide and flecainide are referred to as CAST I while the arm involving moricizine is referred to as CAST II

- all arms of the CAST trial were ultimately stopped early when it became clear that the study medications were associated with increased mortality (although morcizine was not associated with significantly higher mortality in CAST II, data from a preliminary phase showed increased mortality)

Table 1: CAST I's Key Findings

Outcome	Encainide Group	Flecainide Group	Placebo Group	P Value (active drugs vs. placebo)
Death or cardiac arrest due to an arrhythmia	6.7%	4.3%	2.2%	0.0004
Death or cardiac arrest due to all causes	10.2%	5.9%	3.5%	0.0001

Table 2: CAST II's Key Findings

Outcome	Morcizine Group	Placebo Group	P Value
Death or cardiac arrest due to an arrhythmia	9.1%	7.7%	0.40
Death or cardiac arrest due to all causes	16.2%	13.1%	Not reported

Other Relevant Studies and Information:

- The EMIAT[43] and CAMIAT[44] trials evaluated amiodarone for the suppression of ventricular arrhythmias following myocardial infarctions, and although these studies showed a small reduction in deaths due to arrhythmias, there was no all-cause mortality benefit.

- Given the long term side effects of amiodarone, it is only recommended for arrhythmia suppression in a few selected situations. Currently, beta-blockers, and, when appropriate, implantable cardioverter-defibrillators (ICDs), are first-line therapy to prevent arrhythmic deaths in patients following myocardial infarction.

SUMMARY AND IMPLICATIONS:

Although ventricular arrhythmias following a myocardial infarction are associated with cardiac mortality, and although anti-arrhythmic medications can successfully suppress these arrhythmias, the anti-arrhythmic medications used in CAST did not protect patients from cardiac death. In fact, these medications appeared to increase cardiac mortality. Not only did CAST lead to an immediate change in practice (since patients frequently had been receiving anti-arrhythmics following a myocardial infarction), but it also had broader importance: the trial highlighted the need for well-designed clinical trials using placebo controls and hard clinical endpoints prior to the introduction of new therapies.

---

43 Julian et al. Randomised trial of effect of amiodarone on mortality in patients with left-ventricular dysfunction after recent myocardial infarction: European Myocardial Infarct Amiodarone Trial Investigators (EMIAT). Lancet. 1997;349(9053):667-74.

44 Cairns et al. Randomised trial of outcome after myocardial infarction in patients with frequent or repetitive ventricular premature depolarisations: Canadian Amiodarone Myocardial Infarction Arrhythmia Trial Investigators (CAMIAT). Lancet. 1997;349(9053):675-82.

CLINICAL CASE: ARRHYTHMIA SUPPRESSION FOLLOWING MYOCARDIAL INFARCTION

CASE HISTORY:

A 60 year old woman with a history of a myocardial infarction 6 months ago is admitted to the hospital for pneumonia. Incidentally, she is noted to have recurrent short runs of premature ventricular beats (3-5 beats). She does not have any symptoms resulting from the premature beats.

Based on the results of CAST, how should you treat her for these premature beats?

SUGGESTED ANSWER:

CAST suggested that anti-arrhythmic drug therapy may increase mortality in patients with premature ventricular beats following myocardial infarction. Thus, this patient should not receive anti-arrhythmic therapy with the exception of a beta-blocker – which is recommended in all patients following myocardial infarction. In addition, her electrolytes should be checked to make sure there aren't any metabolic disturbances contributing to the premature beats.

CHOOSING FIRST-LINE THERAPY FOR HYPERTENSION:

THE ALLHAT TRIAL[45]

"[The] results of ALLHAT indicate that thiazide-type diuretics should be considered first for pharmacologic therapy in patients with hypertension. They are unsurpassed in lowering [blood pressure], reducing clinical events, and tolerability, and they are less costly."

- The ALLHAT Investigators[45]

Research Question: What is the preferred first-line medication for the treatment of hypertension: thiazide diuretics or any of the more recently developed blood pressure medications?

---

45 ALLHAT Officers and Coordinators for the ALLHAT Collaborative Research Group. Major outcomes in high-risk hypertensive patients randomized to angiotensin-converting enzyme inhibitor or calcium channel blocker vs diuretic: The antihypertensive and lipid-lowering treatment to prevent heart attack trial (ALLHAT). JAMA. 2002 Dec 18;288(23):2981-97.

Funding: The National Heart, Lung, and Blood Institute (NHLBI).

Year Study Began: 1994

Year Study Published: 2002

Study Location: Approximately 600 general medicine and specialty clinics in the U.S., Canada, Puerto Rico, and the Virgin Islands.

Who Was Studied: Adults ≥55 with stage 1 or stage 2 hypertension and at least one additional cardiovascular (CV) risk factor, including prior myocardial infarction or stroke, left ventricular hypertrophy, diabetes type 2, current smoking, HDL cholesterol <35, or known atherosclerosis.

Who Was Excluded: Patients with a history of symptomatic heart failure, those with an ejection fraction <35%, and those with a serum creatinine >2 mg/dl.

How Many Patients: 33,357 (>42,000 patients were originally included, however an arm of the trial involving patients receiving doxazosin was terminated early when it became clear that doxazosin was inferior to other study medications)

Study Overview:

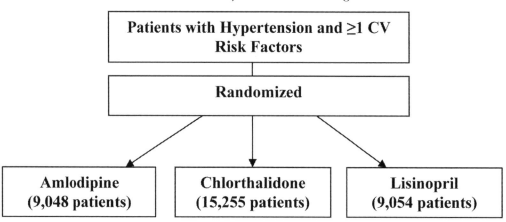

Figure 1: Summary of ALLHAT's Design

- A disproportionate number of patients were assigned to the chlorthalidone arm because medications from this class (thiazide diuretics) were the established first-line treatment for hypertension at the time. Assigning more patients to the chlorthalidone arm allowed for greater statistical power for detecting differences between chlorthalidone and the other study medications.

Study Intervention: Patients were randomly assigned in a double-blinded fashion to receive either a thiazide diuretic (chlorthalidone, initially at a dose of 12.5 mg with a maximum dose of 25 mg); a calcium channel blocker (amlodipine, initially at a dose of 2.5 mg with a maximum dose of 10 mg); or an ACE inhibitor (lisinopril, initially at a dose of 10 mg with a maximum dose of 40 mg).

After being randomized, patients discontinued any prior antihypertensive medications and immediately began taking their assigned medication. The goal blood pressure for all patients was <140/90, and the study medications were titrated as needed to achieve this goal.

When the goal blood pressure could not be achieved with the study medication, additional open-label medications were added (these medications were added similarly in all trial arms).

Follow-Up: Mean of 4.9 years

Endpoints: Primary outcome: a composite of fatal coronary heart disease (CHD) and nonfatal myocardial infarction (MI). Secondary outcomes included: heart failure, stroke, and all-cause mortality.

RESULTS:

- after 5 years, 68.2% of patients in the chlorthalidone group achieved the blood pressure goal vs. 66.3% in the amlodipine group (P=0.09) and 61.2% in the lisinopril group (P<0.001)

Table 1: Summary of ALLHAT's Key Findings[a]

Outcome	Chlorthalidone	Amlodipine	Lisinopril	P Value[b]
Heart failure	7.7%	10.2%	8.7%	<0.001, <0.001
Stroke	5.6%	5.4%	6.3%	0.28, 0.02
All-cause mortality	17.3%	16.8%	17.2%	0.20, 0.90
Fatal CHD and non-fatal MI	11.5%	11.3%	11.4%	0.65, 0.81

[a]Rates are 6-year event rates per 100 persons.
[b]Chlorthalidone vs. amlodipine, chlorthalidone vs. lisinopril.

Criticisms and Limitations: The ALLHAT investigators chose to use chlorthalidone to represent thiazide diuretics since this was the best-studied agent in the class, however the less potent hydrochlorothiazide is more commonly used in the U.S. ALLHAT's findings may not be applicable to hydrochlorothiazide.

Other Relevant Studies and Information:

- An initial arm of ALLHAT involving doxazosin was terminated early when initial data indicated that chlorthalidone reduced the risk of cardiovascular events relative to doxazosin[46].

- The ACCOMPLISH trial compared hydrochlorothiazide vs. amlodipine (both in combination with benazepril) in patients with hypertension and high CV risk and showed amlodipine to be superior[47]. Many experts believe that the discrepancy between the results of ALLHAT and ACCOMPLISH is due to the fact that ALLHAT used chlorthalidone while ACCOMPLISH used hydrochlorothiazide. In addition, the dose of hydrochlorothiazide (12.5 - 25 mg) used in ACCOMPLISH is lower than some experts recommend.

- A recent analysis showed that, despite ALLHAT's finding that chlorthalidone is as effective as amlodipine and lisinopril, the results did not increase the use of thiazide diuretics in the U.S. to the extent that might have been expected[48].

- The Joint National Committee on High Blood Pressure recommends thiazides as first-line agents for hypertension in most patients[49].

SUMMARY AND IMPLICATIONS:

ALLHAT found that chlorthalidone, an inexpensive thiazide diuretic, is at least as effective as – and in some respects superior to – amlodipine

---

46 The ALLHAT Officers and Coordinators for the ALLHAT Collaborative Research Group. Major cardiovascular events in hypertensive patients randomized to doxazosin vs chlorthalidone: the Antihypertensive and Lipid-Lowering Treatment to Prevent Heart Attack Trial (ALLHAT). JAMA. 2000;283:1967-1975.

47 Jamerson et al. Benazepril plus amlodipine or hydrochlorothiazide for hypertension in high-risk patients. N Engl J Med. 2008 Dec 4;359(23):2417-2428.

48 Stafford et al. Impact of the ALLHAT/JNC7 Dissemination Project on Thiazide-Type Diuretic Use. Arch Intern Med. 2010 May 24;170(10):851-8.

49 Chobanian et al. The Seventh Report of the Joint National Committee on Prevention, Detection, Evaluation, and Treatment of High Blood Pressure: the JNC 7 report. JAMA. 2003 May 21;289(19):2560-72.

and lisinopril as first-line therapy in high risk patients with hypertension. Thiazide diuretics remain the recommended first-line medication for patients with hypertension.

CLINICAL CASE: CHOOSING FIRST LINE THERAPY FOR HYPERTENSION

CASE HISTORY:

A 60 year old man with diabetes has been diagnosed with hypertension after repeated blood pressure measurements averaging 162/94. He reports feeling well. Routine laboratory tests are normal, except for the presence of moderate proteinuria.

Based on the results of ALLHAT, how should this patient be treated?

SUGGESTED ANSWER:

ALLHAT established that a thiazide diuretic – chlorthalidone – is at least as effective as several other medications as first-line therapy in high risk patients with hypertension. For this reason, the Joint National Committee (JNC) on High Blood Pressure recommends thiazides as first-line agents for hypertension in most patients.

The patient in this vignette has diabetic nephropathy (due to his proteinuria), however. In such patients, the JNC recommends an angiotensin receptor blocker (ARB) or an ACE inhibitor as first-line treatment for hypertension rather than a thiazide. Still, this patient has stage II hypertension (systolic blood pressure ≥160 or diastolic blood pressure ≥100) for which the JNC recommends two medications as initial therapy. Thus, this patient should be started on both a thiazide diuretic (many experts believe that chlorthalidone is superior to hydrochlorothiazide) as well as an ARB or ACE inhibitor.

STATINS IN HEALTHY PATIENTS WITH AN ELEVATED C-REACTIVE PROTEIN:

THE JUPITER TRIAL[50]

"In this randomized trial of [healthy patients] with elevated levels of high-sensitivity C-reactive protein, rosuvastatin significantly reduced the incidence of major cardiovascular events, despite the fact that nearly all study participants had [normal lipid levels]."

- Ridker et al.[50]

Research Question: Are statins effective in healthy patients with elevated C-reactive protein levels but without hyperlipidema?

---

50 Ridker et al. Rosuvastatin to prevent vascular events in men and women with elevated C-reactive protein. N Engl J Med. 2008 Nov 20;359(21):2195-2207.

Funding: AstraZeneca.

Year Study Began: 2003

Year Study Published: 2008

Study Location: 1,315 sites in 26 countries

Who Was Studied: Men ≥50 and women ≥60 without prior cardiovascular disease and with an LDL cholesterol <130 mg/dl and a high-sensitivity C-reactive protein (CRP) ≥2.0 mg/l. The median CRP of patients screened for the trial was 1.9 mg/l (i.e. slightly more than half of all screened patients had a CRP below the level necessary for trial inclusion).

Who Was Excluded: Patients with a triglyceride level ≥500, those with previous or current use of lipid-lowering medications, those with an elevated alanine aminotransferase, creatine kinase, or creatinine, those with diabetes or un-controlled hypertension, and those with cancer in the five years prior to enrollment. In addition, patients who did not take more than 80% of pre-scribed placebo pills in a four-week pilot study were excluded since these patients were unlikely to comply with the trial medications.

How Many Patients: 17,802

Study Overview:

Figure 1: Summary of JUPITER's Design

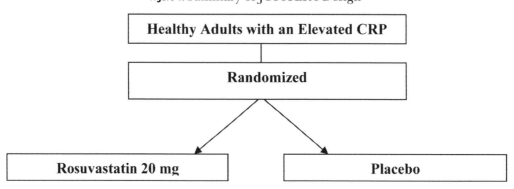

Study Intervention: Patients were randomly assigned to receive either rosuvas-tatin 20 mg daily or placebo.

Follow-Up: Median 1.9 years

Endpoints: Primary outcome: a composite of nonfatal myocardial infarctions, nonfatal strokes, hospitalizations for unstable angina, arterial revasculariza-tion, or cardiovascular death. Secondary outcome: death from any cause.

RESULTS:

- at baseline, the median LDL was 108 mg/dl in both groups; after 12 months, the median LDL was 55 mg/dl in the rosuvastatin group vs. 110 mg/dl in the placebo group

- at baseline, the median CRP was 4.2 mg/l in the rosuvastatin group and 4.3 mg/l in the placebo group; after 12 months, the median CRP was 2.2 mg/l in the rosuvastatin group vs. 3.5 mg/dl in the placebo group

Table 1: JUPITER's Key Findings[a]

Outcome	Rosuvastatin Group	Placebo Group	P Value
Primary composite outcome	0.77	1.36	<0.00001
Myocardial infarctions	0.17	0.37	0.0002
Stroke	0.18	0.34	0.002
Death	1.00	1.25	0.02

[a]Event rates are per 100 person-years, i.e. the number of events that occurred for every 100 years of participant time. For example, 0.77 events per 100 person-years means that there were, on average, 0.77 events among 50 subjects who were each enrolled in the trial for two years.

- the incidence of diabetes was slightly higher during the study period in the rosuvastatin group than in the placebo group (3.0% vs. 2.4%, P=0.01)

Criticisms and Limitations: The absolute benefits of rosuvastatin were small: 95 patients would need to be treated for two years to prevent one cardiovascular event. Therefore, it is debatable whether the benefits of statins in healthy patients with an elevated CRP outweigh the potential long-term side effects.

In addition, it is unclear whether CRP levels should be used to help determine which patients should be treated with statins. It is possible that patients with normal CRP levels benefit just as much from statins as those with elevated levels.

Other Relevant Studies and Information:

- Other trials have also suggested a benefit of statins in patients without known cardiovascular disease, however the absolute benefits of statins among such patients are very small[51,52]

- Guidelines from the Centers for Disease Control and the American Heart Association, among other organizations, indicate that CRP measurement may be considered among patients with an intermediate cardiovascular risk (10%-20% over 10 years) to help determine whether or not statins should be used[53]. However, guidelines from the United States Preventive Services Task Force do not recommend measuring CRP levels to help assess cardiovascular risk[54]

SUMMARY AND IMPLICATIONS:

Statin therapy reduced cardiovascular events in healthy patients with elevated CRP levels and normal lipids, however the absolute benefits of statin therapy were small. The study did not assess whether CRP measurement is important for determining which patients should receive statins.

---

51 Taylor et al. Statins for the primary prevention of cardiovascular disease. Cochrane Database Syst Rev. 2011.

52 Ray et al. Statins and all-cause mortality in high-risk primary prevention: a meta-analysis of 11 randomized controlled trials involving 65,229 participants. Arch Intern Med. 2010;170(12):1024.

53 Pearson et al. Markers of inflammation and cardiovascular disease: application to clinical and public health practice: A statement for healthcare professionals from the Centers for Disease Control and Prevention and the American Heart Association. Circulation. 2003;107(3):499.

54 U.S. Preventive Services Task Force. Using nontraditional risk factors in coronary heart disease risk assessment: U.S. Preventive Services Task Force recommendation statement. Ann Intern Med. 2009;151(7):474.

CLINICAL CASE: STATINS IN HEALTHY PATIENTS WITH AN ELEVATED C-REACTIVE PROTEIN

CASE HISTORY:

A 70 year old woman with a history of hypertension and tobacco use visits your clinic for a routine visit. She has a total cholesterol of 180, an HDL of 48, and an LDL of 120. Based on the results of JUPITER, should you measure her CRP to help assess her cardiovascular risk? If her CRP is elevated, should she be started on a statin?

SUGGESTED ANSWER:

JUPITER demonstrated a small but significant benefit of statin therapy among patients with a CRP ≥2.0 mg/l. Since only patients with an elevated CRP level were included, the study did not assess whether CRP measurement is important for determining which patients should receive statins.

Guidelines from the United States Preventive Services Task Force (USPSTF) do not recommend measuring CRP levels to assess cardiovascular risk. However, guidelines from the Centers for Disease Control and the American Heart Association (CDC/AHA) indicate that CRP measurement may be considered among patients with an intermediate cardiovascular risk (10%-20% over 10 years) to help determine whether statins should be used. If the CRP is measured, it may assist in treatment decisions (e.g. whether or not to institute statin therapy).

The patient in this vignette is at intermediate cardiovascular risk (10-year Framingham risk score is approximately 10% based on the risk factors described above). If you chose to follow the CDC/AHA guidelines, you might measure her CRP and initiate statin therapy if the level is elevated. However, you could also follow the USPSTF guidelines and opt not to check the CRP.

RATE VS. RHYTHM CONTROL FOR ATRIAL FIBRILLATION:

THE AFFIRM TRIAL[55]

"[In older patients with atrial fibrillation and cardiovascular risk factors] the strategy of restoring and maintaining sinus rhythm [has] no clear advantage over the strategy of controlling the ventricular rate ..."

- The AFFIRM Investigators[55]

Research Question: Should patients with atrial fibrillation be managed with a strategy of rate-control or rhythm-control?

Funding: The National Heart, Lung, and Blood Institute.

Year Study Began: 1997

Year Study Published: 2002

---

55 The AFFIRM Investigators. A comparison of rate control and rhythm control in patients with atrial fibrillation. N Engl J Med. 2002 Dec 5;347(23):1825-33.

Study Location: 200 sites in the U.S. and Canada

Who Was Studied: Adults with atrial fibrillation who were at least 65 or who had other risk factors for stroke. In addition, only patients likely to have recurrent atrial fibrillation requiring long-term treatment were eligible.

Who Was Excluded: Patients in whom anticoagulation was contraindicated.

How Many Patients: 4,060

Study Overview:

Figure 1: Summary of AFFIRM's Design

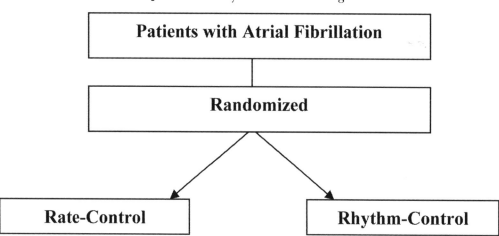

Study Intervention: Patients in the rhythm-control group received antiarrhythmic drugs (most commonly amiodarone and/or sotalol) at the discretion of the treating physician. If needed, physicians could attempt to cardiovert patients to sinus rhythm. Anticoagulation with warfarin was encouraged, but could be stopped at the physician's discretion if the patient remained in sinus rhythm for at least 4 (and preferably 12) consecutive weeks.

Patients in the rate-control group received beta-blockers, calcium-channel blockers, or digoxin at the discretion of the treating physician. The target heart rate was ≤80 beats per minute at rest and ≤110 beats per minute during a six-minute walk test. All patients in the rate-control group received anticoagulation with warfarin.

Follow-Up: Mean of 3.5 years

Endpoints: Primary outcome: All-cause mortality. Secondary outcomes: A composite of death, disabling stroke, disabling anoxic encephalopathy, major bleeding, and cardiac arrest; and hospitalizations.

RESULTS:

- in the rate-control group, at the five-year visit, 34.6% of patients were in sinus rhythm and over 80% of those in atrial fibrillation had adequate heart rate control

- in the rhythm-control group, at the five-year visit, 62.6% of patients were in sinus rhythm

- after five years, 14.9% of patients in the rate-control group crossed over to the rhythm-control group, most commonly due to symptoms such as palpitations or episodes of heart failure

- after five years, 37.5% of patients in the rhythm-control group crossed over to the rate-control group, most commonly due to an inability to maintain sinus rhythm or due to drug intolerance

- throughout the study, more than 85% of patients in the rate-control group were taking warfarin compared to approximately 70% of patients in the rhythm-control group; most strokes in both groups occurred among patients not receiving a therapeutic dose of warfarin

Table 1: Summary of AFFIRM's Key Findings

Outcome	Rate-control Group	Rhythm-control Group	P Value
All-cause mortality	25.9%	26.7%	0.08
Composite of death, disabling stroke, disabling anoxic encephalopathy, major bleeding, and cardiac arrest	32.7%	32.0%	0.33
Hospitalizations	73.0%	80.1%	<0.001

Criticisms and Limitations: The trial did not include young patients without cardiovascular risk factors, especially those with paroxysmal atrial fibrillation, and therefore the results may not apply to these patients.

In addition, approximately half of the patients in the study had symptomatic episodes of atrial fibrillation less than once a month. It is possible that patients with more frequent or persistent symptoms would derive a benefit from rhythm-control.

Other Relevant Studies and Information:

• A number of smaller randomized trials comparing rate-control and rhythm-control in patients with atrial fibrillation have come to similar conclusions as AFFIRM[56,57,58,59]

• Trials comparing rate-control vs. rhythm-control in patients with atrial fibrillation and heart failure have also failed to show a benefit of rhythm-control[60,61]

SUMMARY AND IMPLICATIONS:

In high risk patients with atrial fibrillation, a strategy of rate-control is at least as effective as a strategy of rhythm-control. Rhythm-control does not appear to obviate the need for anticoagulation. Because the medications used for rate control are usually safer than those used for rhythm control, rate-control is the preferred strategy for treating most high risk patients with atrial fibrillation. These findings do not necessarily apply to younger patients without cardiovascular risk factors who were not included in AFFIRM, however.

---

56 Van Gelder IC et al. A comparison of rate control and rhythm control in patients with recurrent persistent atrial fibrillation. N Engl J Med. 2002;347(23):1834-40.

57 Hohnloser SH et al. Rhythm or rate control in atrial fibrillation–Pharmacological Intervention in Atrial Fibrillation (PIAF): a randomised trial. Lancet. 2000;356(9244):1789-94.

58 Carlsson J et al. Randomized trial of rate-control vs. rhythm-control in persistent atrial fibrillation: the Strategies of Treatment of Atrial Fibrillation (STAF) study. J Am Coll Cardiol. 2003;41(10):1690-6.

59 Opolski G et al. Rate control vs rhythm control in patients with nonvalvular persistent atrial fibrillation: the results of the Polish How to Treat Chronic Atrial Fibrillation (HOT CAFE) Study. Chest. 2004;126(2):476-86.

60 Roy D et al. Rhythm control vs. rate control for atrial fibrillation and heart failure. N Engl J Med. 2008;358(25):2667-77.

61 Kober et al. Increased mortality after dronedarone therapy for severe heart failure. N Engl J Med. 2008;358(25):2678-87.

CLINICAL CASE: RATE VS. RHYTHM CONTROL IN ATRIAL FIBRILLATION

CASE HISTORY:

A 75 year old woman with diabetes and hypertension is noted on routine examination to have an irregular heart rate of approximately 120 beats per minute. She denies chest pain, shortness of breath, and other concerning symptoms. An EKG confirms a diagnosis of atrial fibrillation.

Based on the results of AFFIRM, how should this patient be treated?

SUGGESTED ANSWER:

AFFIRM showed that rate-control is at least as effective as rhythm-control for managing atrial fibrillation. Because the medications used for rate control are usually safer than those used for rhythm control, rate-control is generally the preferred strategy for managing the condition.

The patient in this vignette is typical of patients included in AFFIRM. Thus, she should be treated initially with a rate-control strategy (beta-blockers are frequently used as first-line agents). In the unlikely event that this patient's heart rate could not be controlled or if she were to develop bothersome symptoms that did not improve with a rate-control strategy, rhythm-control might be considered. In addition, this patient should receive anticoagulation to reduce her risk for stroke.

LENIENT VS. STRICT HEART RATE CONTROL FOR ATRIAL FIBRILLATION:

THE RACE II TRIAL[62]

"[For] both patients and health care providers, lenient rate control is [as effective and] more convenient [than strict rate control in patients with atrial fibrillation] ..."

- Van Gelder et al.[62]

Research Question: Should the heart rate target in patients with atrial fibrillation be strict (<80 beats per minute) or lenient (<110 beats per minute)?

Funding: The Netherlands Heart Foundation, as well as unrestricted educational grants from several pharmaceutical companies.

Year Study Began: 2005

62 Van Gelder et al. Lenient vs. strict rate control in patients with atrial fibrillation. N Engl J Med. 2010 Apr 15;362(15):1363-73.

Year Study Published: 2010

Study Location: 33 centers in the Netherlands

Who Was Studied: Patients with permanent atrial fibrillation (i.e. longstanding) and a mean resting heart rate >80 beats per minute.

Who Was Excluded: Patients over the age of 80, those with unstable heart failure, and those unable to exercise.

How Many Patients: 614

Study Overview:

Figure 1: Summary of RACE II's Design

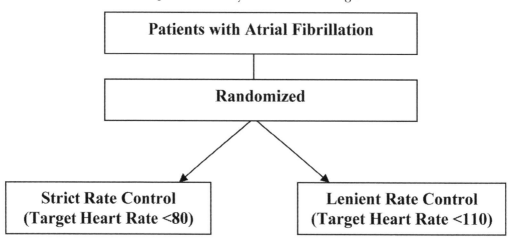

Study Intervention: Patients in the strict rate control group had a heart rate target of <80 beats per minute at rest and <110 beats per minute with moderate exercise. Patients in the lenient rate control group had a resting heart rate target of <110 beats per minute.

Patients in both groups received beta-blockers, nondihydropyridine calcium-channel blockers (e.g. diltiazem), and digoxin. These medications were titrated at the physician's discretion to achieve the target heart rate. Patients were evaluated every 2 weeks until the targets were achieved.

When the target heart rate could not be achieved or when symptoms could not be controlled, patients could receive electrical cardioversion or ablation at the discretion of their physicians.

Follow-Up: At least 2 years and a maximum of 3 years

Endpoints: Primary outcome: A composite of death from cardiovascular causes, hospitalizations for heart failure, stroke, systemic embolism, major bleeding, syncope, sustained ventricular tachycardia, cardiac arrest, life-threatening medication complications, and implantation of a pacemaker or cardioverter-defibrillator.

Statistical Note: The trial was designed to assess the non-inferiority of a lenient strategy compared to a strict strategy, i.e. that a lenient strategy is not appreciably worse than a strict strategy.

RESULTS:

- after the dose adjustment period, the mean resting heart rate was 93 beats per minute in the lenient group vs. 76 beats per minute in the strict group (P<0.001)

- symptoms associated with atrial fibrillation were similar in both groups

- patients in the lenient group required fewer physician visits and fewer medications to achieve the heart rate target

- 10.3% of patients in the lenient group vs. 1.0% in the strict group required no medications to achieve the heart rate targets (P<0.001)

Table 1: Summary of RACE II's Key Findings[a]

Outcome	Lenient Group	Strict Group	P Value
Composite primary outcome	12.9%	14.9%	0.001 for non-inferiority[b]
All-cause mortality	5.6%	6.6%	Non-significant[c]
Cardiovascular mortality	2.9%	3.9%	Non-significant[c]
Heart failure hospitalizations	3.8%	4.1%	Non-significant[c]

[a]Percentages are estimated 3-year cumulative incidences
[b]This p-value is for the non-inferiority analysis, i.e. lenient control was non-inferior to strict control at a p-value of 0.001
[c]Actual p-value not reported

Criticisms and Limitations: Patients in RACE II were only followed for 2-3 years and it is possible that the benefits of a strict rate control strategy take longer than this to become apparent.

No other well designed trials have compared different heart rate targets in patients with atrial fibrillation. Other trials should be conducted to confirm RACE II's findings.

SUMMARY AND IMPLICATIONS:

A lenient heart rate target of <110 beats per minute at rest is as effective as a strict target of <80 beats per minute in patients with permanent atrial fibrillation. The lenient target is more convenient and requires the use of fewer medications.

CLINICAL CASE: LENIENT VS. STRICT RATE CONTROL FOR ATRIAL FIBRILLATION

CASE HISTORY:

A 76 year old woman with atrial fibrillation, diabetes, coronary artery disease, and hypertension presents to your office for a regular visit. She is on 9 medications, including metoprolol and diltiazem to control her atrial fibrillation. She feels well, but reports that it is very difficult to take all of her medications each day. In addition, some of the medications make her "feel funny." On exam, she is well-appearing, has a heart rate of 70, and a blood pressure of 116/72.

Based on the results of RACE II, how might you adjust her medications?

SUGGESTED ANSWER:

RACE II found that a lenient heart rate target of <110 beats per minute at rest is as effective as a strict target of <80 beats per minute in patients with permanent atrial fibrillation. The lenient target is more convenient and requires the use of fewer medications.

The patient in this vignette is typical of patients included in RACE II. Thus, a resting heart rate target of <110 could be considered for her. She is on both a beta-blocker and a nondihydropyridine calcium channel blocker – a combination that may lead to bradycardia and hypotension and might explain why she feels "funny" at times. Based on the results of RACE II, you might discontinue her diltiazem and monitor her response (i.e. reassess her in a few days to recheck her heart rate and blood pressure and assess whether the "funny feeling" that she gets has improved). Because this patient has coronary artery disease, she should be continued on the metoprolol.

BETA-BLOCKERS FOR SYSTOLIC HEART FAILURE:

THE MERIT-HF TRIAL[63,64]

"In this study of patients with symptomatic [systolic] heart failure, [extended release metoprolol] improved survival, reduced the need for hospitalizations due to worsening heart failure … and had beneficial effects on patient well-being."

- Hjalmarson et al.[63]

Research Question: Should patients with chronic systolic heart failure receive beta-blockers?

Funding: AstraZeneca.

63 Hjalmarson et al. Effects of controlled-release metoprolol on total mortality, hospitalizations, and well-being in patients with heart failure: The metoprolol CR/XL randomized intervention trial in congestive heart failure. JAMA. 2000;283(10):1295-1302.

64 MERIT-HF Study Group. Effect of metoprolol CR/XL in chronic heart failure: Metoprolol CR/XL Randomised Intervention Trial in Congestive Heart Failure (MERIT-HF). Lancet. 1999 Jun 12;353(9169):2001-7.

Year Study Began: 1997

Year Study Published: 1999 and 2000

Study Location: 313 sites in 14 countries

Who Was Studied: Adults 40-80 with symptomatic chronic heart failure and an ejection fraction ≤40%. In addition, patients were required to have symptoms corresponding to New York Heart Association (NYHA) class II – IV (class II corresponds to mild symptoms and slight limitations with ordinary activities, while class IV corresponds to severe symptoms with impairment at rest). Patients also were required to have a resting heart rate ≥68 and to be receiving other appropriate therapy for heart failure (e.g. diuretics and an ACE inhibitor).

Who Was Excluded: Patients with a myocardial infarction or unstable angina in the 28 days prior to enrollment, those with decompensated heart failure (e.g. pulmonary edema or signs of hypoperfusion), and those with a supine systolic blood pressure <100 mm Hg.

How Many Patients: 3,991

Study Overview:

Figure 1: Summary of MERIT-HF's Design

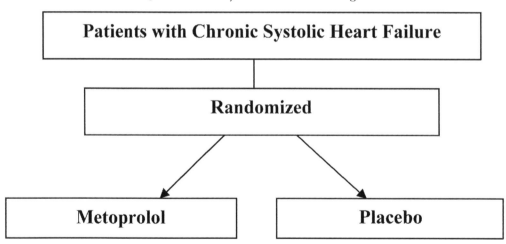

Study Intervention: Patients assigned to the metoprolol group received metoprolol controlled-release/extended release (CR/XL), initially at a dose of 25 mg once per day in patients with NYHA class II heart failure or 12.5 mg once per day in patients with NYHA class III – IV heart failure. Every two weeks, the dose was doubled until the target dose of 200 mg daily was reached. If patients did not tolerate the dose increase, the regimen could be modified.

Patients assigned to the placebo group received placebo according to the same protocol.

Follow-Up: Mean of 1 year (2.4 years was planned, but the trial was stopped early when it became clear that metoprolol CR/XL was effective)

Endpoints: Primary outcomes: All-cause mortality and a composite of all-cause mortality and hospitalizations. Secondary outcomes: hospitalizations due to heart failure; change in NYHA class as assessed by physicians; and quality of life and symptom scores as assessed by patients on the Minnesota Living with Heart Failure questionnaire and the McMaster Overall Treatment Evaluation (OTE) questionnaire.

RESULTS:

- the trial was stopped early when it became clear that patients receiving metoprolol had better outcomes than those in the placebo group

- the mean age of study subjects was 64, the mean ejection fraction was 28%, and 55% of patients had NYHA class III heart failure

- 64% of patients reached the target metoprolol dose of 200 mg per day (the rest did not tolerate higher doses)

Table 1: Summary of the MERIT-HF's Key Findings[a]

Outcome	Metoprolol Group	Control Group	P Value
All-cause mortality	7.2%	11.0%	0.00009
Hospitalizations			
Total	29.1%	33.3%	<0.001
Due to heart failure	10.0%	14.7%	<0.001
All-cause mortality and hospitalizations	32.2%	38.3%	<0.001

[a]Rates are per year of patient follow-up.

- metoprolol had a modestly positive impact on the NYHA class (P=0.003 for the trend): for example 28.6% of patients in the metoprolol group vs. 25.8% of patients in the placebo group improved at least one NYHA class during the study period

- the OTE quality of life and symptom scores were significantly higher in the metoprolol group than in the placebo group (P=0.009), however quality of life and symptom scores on the Living with Heart Failure questionnaire were not significantly different between the groups

- dizziness, bradycardia, and hypotension were slightly more common in the metoprolol group, but otherwise adverse effects were generally more common in the placebo group

Criticisms and Limitations: This trial excluded patients with an ejection fraction >40% as well as those with a recent myocardial infarction or unstable angina.

Other Relevant Studies and Information:

- Other studies have also demonstrated the benefits of beta-blockers, including carvedilol[65,66,67,68,69] and bisoprolol[70], in patients with chronic systolic heart failure (carvedilol blocks beta-1, beta-2, and alpha-1 receptors while bisoprolol and metoprolol are beta-1 selective)

- The COMET trial[71], which directly compared carvedilol with short-acting metoprolol in patients with chronic systolic heart failure, showed carvedilol to be superior, however the metoprolol dose may have been too small in COMET; in addition, MERIT-HF used controlled

---

65 Packer et al. Double-blind, placebo-controlled study of the effects of carvedilol in patients with moderate to severe heart failure. The PRECISE Trial. Prospective Randomized Evaluation of Carvedilol on Symptoms and Exercise. Circulation. 1996;94(11):2793.

66 Colucci et al. Carvedilol inhibits clinical progression in patients with mild symptoms of heart failure. US Carvedilol Heart Failure Study Group. Circulation. 1996;94(11):2800.

67 Bristow et al. Carvedilol produces dose-related improvements in left ventricular function and survival in subjects with chronic heart failure. MOCHA Investigators. Circulation. 1996;94(11):2807.

68 Packer et al. The effect of carvedilol on morbidity and mortality in patients with chronic heart failure. U.S. Carvedilol Heart Failure Study Group. N Engl J Med. 1996;334(21):1349.

69 Packer et al. Effect of carvedilol on survival in severe chronic heart failure. N Engl J Med. 2001;344(22):1651.

70 The Cardiac Insufficiency Bisoprolol Study II (CIBIS-II): a randomised trial. Lancet. 1999;353(9146):9.

71 Poole-Wilson PA. Comparison of carvedilol and metoprolol on clinical outcomes in patients with chronic heart failure in the Carvedilol or Metoprolol European Trial (COMET): randomised controlled trial. Lancet. 2003;362(9377):7.

release/extended release metoprolol while COMET used short-acting metoprolol

- There are no high-quality studies demonstrating the efficacy of beta-blockers in patients with diastolic heart failure

SUMMARY AND IMPLICATIONS:

Metoprolol CR/XL reduced mortality, prevented hospitalizations, and improved symptoms and quality of life in patients with chronic systolic heart failure. Beta-blockers are now a standard part of care for such patients.

CLINICAL CASE: BETA-BLOCKERS FOR SYSTOLIC HEART FAILURE

CASE HISTORY:

A 78 year old woman with chronic heart failure visits your office for evaluation. She has had hypertension for as long as she can remember. The patient is able to ambulate short distances, but she must stop every 10 feet to catch her breath (NYHA class III). A recent echocardiogram reveals an ejection fraction of 45-50% with evidence of moderate diastolic dysfunction. Her medications include lisinopril and furosemide.

On exam, the patient's heart rate is 78 and her blood pressure is 158/96. She has jugular venous distension and lower extremity edema.

Based on the results of MERIT-HF, should you add a beta-blocker to her regimen?

SUGGESTED ANSWER:

The MERIT-HF trial – and other trials of beta-blockers in chronic heart failure – demonstrated that beta-blockers are effective in patients with systolic dysfunction. In most of these trials, patients had an ejection fraction ≤40%. No high quality trials have demonstrated the benefit of beta-blockers in diastolic dysfunction.

The patient in this vignette has chronic heart failure with a combination of systolic and diastolic dysfunction, but would not have been included in MERIT-HF because her ejection fraction is >40%. The benefits of beta-blockers in patients with diastolic heart failure have never been proven. Still, because her heart rate and blood pressure are elevated, it might be reasonable to initiate a beta-blocker and monitor her response closely. It would also be reasonable to withhold treatment because of the lack of evidence, however.

INITIAL TREATMENT OF STABLE CORONARY ARTERY DISEASE:

THE COURAGE TRIAL[72]

"Our findings [confirm] … that [percutaneous coronary intervention] can be safely deferred in patients with stable coronary artery disease, even in those with extensive, multivessel involvement and inducible ischemia, provided that intensive, multifaceted medical therapy is instituted and maintained."

- Boden et al.[72]

Research Question: Should patients with stable coronary artery disease (CAD) be managed initially with medical therapy vs. percutaneous coronary intervention (PCI)?

---

72 Boden et al. Optimal medical therapy with or without PCI for stable coronary disease. N Engl J Med. 2007 Apr 12;356(15):1503-16.

Funding: The Department of Veterans Affairs and the Canadian Institutes of Health Research.

Year Study Began: 1999

Year Study Published: 2007

Study Location: 50 centers in the U.S. and Canada

Who Was Studied: Adults with stable coronary artery disease as defined by either a ≥70% stenosis in at least one proximal coronary artery along with objective evidence of ischemia on an EKG or stress test; or a ≥80% stenosis in a proximal coronary artery and classic angina symptoms. Patients with multi-vessel disease were included.

Who Was Excluded: Patients with class IV angina, a markedly positive stress test (i.e. substantial ST depression or hypotension during stage 1 of Bruce protocol stress test), refractory heart failure, ejection fraction <30%, or coronary anatomy unsuitable for PCI.

How Many Patients: 2,287

Study Overview:

Figure 1: Summary of COURAGE's Design

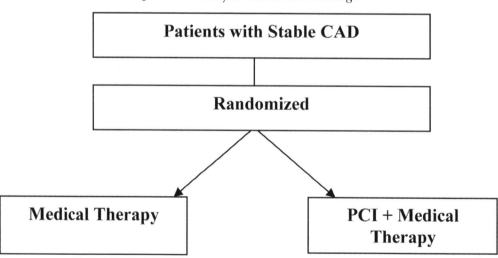

Study Interventions: Patients in the medical therapy group received aspirin (or clopidogrel in patients with an aspirin allergy), lisinopril or losartan, and the following anti-ischemic medications: metoprolol, amlodipine, and isosorbide mononitrate, alone or in combination. In addition, patients received simvastatin alone or in combination with ezetimibe for a goal LDL of 60-85, a goal HDL >40, and a goal triglycerides <150.

Patients in the PCI group underwent target lesion PCI along with additional revascularization as clinically appropriate. Patients in this group also received aspirin and clopidogrel, and the same anti-ischemic medications, blood pressure medications, and lipid management as patients in the medical therapy group.

Follow-Up: Median 4.6 years

Endpoints: Primary outcome: a composite of death from any cause and non-fatal myocardial infarction. Secondary outcomes: angina symptom control and quality of life[73].

RESULTS:

- 88% of patients in the PCI group successfully received stents

- 70% of subjects in both groups achieved an LDL <85, while 65% achieved a systolic blood pressure <130

- initially, patients in the PCI group had a small but significant improvement in angina symptoms and quality of life, however these differences were no longer present by the end of the study period

Table 1: Summary of COURAGE's Key Findings[a]

Outcome	Medical Therapy Group	PCI Group	P Value
Death or non-fatal myocardial infarction	18.5%	19.0%	0.62
Hospitalizations for acute coronary syndrome	11.8%	12.4%	0.56
Additional revascularization necessary[b]	32.6%	21.1%	<0.001

[a]Estimated 4.6-year cumulative event rates
[b]The need for PCI and/or coronary artery bypass surgery in the medical therapy group or the need for a repeat of these procedures in the PCI group.

---

73 Reported in a separate publication: Weintraub et al. Effect of PCI on quality of life in patients with stable coronary disease. N Engl J Med 2008; 358:677.

Criticisms and Limitations: Drug-eluting stents – which now are in common use – were not used in the PCI group until the final six months of the study. Some argue that COURAGE should be repeated using drug-eluting stents (though it is not clear that drug-eluting stents lead to better outcomes than do bare metal stents).

Other Relevant Studies and Information:

- Other studies comparing PCI with medical therapy have come to similar conclusions as the COURAGE trial[74,75].

- The BARI-2D trial showed similar outcomes among patients with diabetes who were treated with medical therapy vs. revascularization (either PCI or coronary artery bypass surgery at their physician's discretion), though a subgroup analysis suggested that patients who received coronary artery bypass surgery had the best outcomes[76].

- The STICH trial, which compared coronary-artery bypass surgery vs. medical therapy in patients with coronary artery disease and an ejection fraction ≤35%, found that the two treatments led to similar mortality rates[77]

- Despite the results of the COURAGE trial, many U.S. patients with stable coronary disease do not receive a trial of optimal medical therapy before undergoing PCI[78].

SUMMARY AND IMPLICATIONS:

In patients with stable coronary artery disease (including multi-vessel disease) medical therapy and percutaneous coronary intervention (PCI) lead to similar outcomes. For most patients, medical therapy is

---

74 Tirkalinos et al. Percutaneous coronary interventions for non-acute coronary artery disease: a quantitative 20-year synopsis and a network meta-analysis. Lancet. 2009;373(9667):911.

75 Stergiopoulos K and Brown DL. Initial coronary stent implantation with medical therapy vs. medical therapy alone for stable coronary artery disease: meta-analysis of randomized controlled trials. *Arch Intern Med.* 2012;172(2):ira110003312-319.

76 BARI 2D Study Group. A randomized trial of therapies for type 2 diabetes and coronary artery disease. N Engl J Med. 2009 Jun 11;360(24):2503-15.

77 Velazquez et al. Coronary-artery bypass surgery in patients with left ventricular dysfunction. NEJM. 2011;364:1607-16.

78 Boden et al. Patterns and intensity of medical therapy in patients undergoing percutaneous coronary intervention. JAMA. 2011 May 11;305(18):1882-9.

an appropriate – and generally preferable – initial management strategy, though a substantial proportion of medically managed patients may ultimately require PCI to treat refractory symptoms. Certain high-risk patients, such as those with severe symptoms, may still benefit from initial PCI.

CLINICAL CASE: INITIAL TREATMENT OF STABLE CORONARY ARTERY DISEASE

CASE HISTORY:

A 62 year old man visits your clinic to review the results of his recent stress test. For the past year, he has noted substernal discomfort when climbing steps or walking up hills. The pain is relieved with rest. Aside from a daily baby aspirin, your patient does not take any medications.

During the stress test, your patient was able to exercise for 6 minutes and achieved 7 METS of activity. His peak heart rate was 148 beats per minute. Towards the end of the test, he developed the same substernal chest discomfort that he typically experiences. He also developed lateral ST depressions on EKG. A repeat stress test with nuclear imaging confirmed reversible ischemia in the territory of the left circumflex coronary artery. In addition, the cardiac function appeared to be mildly impaired (ejection fraction 45-50%).

You explain to your patient that he has stable coronary artery disease. Based on the results of the COURAGE trial, how would you treat him?

SUGGESTED ANSWER:

The COURAGE trial suggests that, for most patients with stable coronary artery disease, medical therapy is an appropriate – and generally preferable – initial management strategy.

The patient in this vignette is typical of those included in the COURAGE trial. He doesn't have any of the high risk features that might suggest that he would benefit from immediate revascularization. Thus he would be a good candidate for medical management. Should his symptoms worsen in the future despite optimal medical therapy, he might require revascularization to help manage his symptoms, however revascularization is not necessary at this point.

TREATING ELEVATED BLOOD SUGAR LEVELS IN PATIENTS WITH TYPE 2 DIABETES:

THE UNITED KINGDOM PROSPECTIVE DIABETES STUDY (UKPDS)[79,80]

"UKPDS shows that an intensive glucose-control treatment policy that maintains… [a median hemoglobin A1C of 7.0% - 7.4%] substantially reduces the frequency of [diabetes-related complications]."

- The UKPDS Study Group[79]

79 UK Prospective Diabetes Study Group. Intensive blood-glucose control with sulphonyl-ureas or insulin compared with conventional treatment and risk of complications in patients with type 2 diabetes (UKPDS 33). Lancet. 1998 Sep 12;352(9131):837-53.

80 UK Prospective Diabetes Study Group. Effect of intensive blood-glucose control with metformin on complications in overweight patients with type 2 diabetes (UKPDS 34). Lancet. 1998 Sep 12;352(9131):854-65.

Research Question: Does treating type 2 diabetes with medications to lower the blood sugar reduce diabetes-related complications more than dietary therapy alone?

Funding: The United Kingdom Medical Research Council and other public funding agencies from the United Kingdom; the United States National Institutes of Health; several charitable organizations; and several pharmaceutical companies.

Year Study Began: 1977

Year Study Published: 1998

Study Location: Patients were referred from numerous general practitioner clinics in the United Kingdom.

Who Was Studied: Patients 25-65 with newly diagnosed type 2 diabetes. Patients were required to have a fasting plasma glucose >108 mg/dl on two mornings, 1-3 weeks apart.

Who Was Excluded: Patients with a serum creatinine >2.0 mg/dl, those with a myocardial infarction within the previous year, those with angina or heart failure, those with retinopathy requiring laser treatment, and those with a concurrent illness limiting life expectancy.

How Many Patients: 4,209

Study Overview:

A group of 2,505 patients (both overweight and non-overweight) were randomized to receive either intensive treatment with insulin or a sulphonylurea, or to dietary therapy alone. A group of 1,704 overweight patients were randomized to receive either intensive treatment with metformin, intensive treatment with insulin or a sulphonylurea, or to dietary therapy alone. Figure 1 summarizes the treatment allocation:

Figure 1: Summary of UKPDS's Design

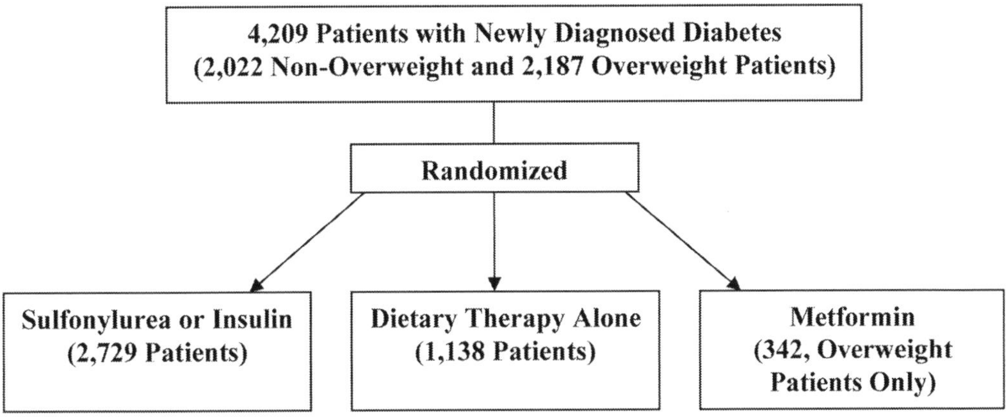

4,209 Patients with Newly Diagnosed Diabetes
(2,022 Non-Overweight and 2,187 Overweight Patients)

Randomized

| **Sulfonylurea or Insulin** **(2,729 Patients)** | **Dietary Therapy Alone** **(1,138 Patients)** | **Metformin** **(342, Overweight Patients Only)** |

Study Intervention:

Patients in the dietary therapy group received counseling from a dietician. Patients in the sulfonylurea/insulin group and in the metformin group received both counseling and medications.

All medications were titrated for a target fasting blood glucose of <108 mg/dl. Patients in the insulin group were initially started on basal insulin, and prandial insulin was added if the daily dose was >14 units or if the pre-meal or bedtime glucose was >126 mg/dl. Patients in the sulphonylurea group received chlorpropamide, glibenclamide, or glipizide. Patients in the metformin group were started on metformin 850 mg once daily, which could be increased to a maximum of 1700 mg in the morning and 850 mg at night.

Patients in the dietary, sulfonylurea, and metformin groups who developed symptoms of hyperglycemia (thirst or polyuria) or who had glucose levels >270 mg/dl were started on additional medications.

Follow-Up: A median of 10.0 years in the sulfonylurea-insulin group and 10.7 years in the metformin group.

Endpoints:

1) Diabetes-related endpoints: sudden death, death from hyperglycemia or hypoglycemia, myocardial infarction, angina, heart failure, stroke, renal failure, amputation, and ophthalmologic complications
2) Diabetes-related deaths: sudden death or death due to myocardial infarction, peripheral vascular disease, renal disease, hyperglycemia, or hypoglycemia
3) All-cause mortality

4) Microvascular disease: vitreous hemorrhage, retinal photocoagulation, or renal failure

---

RESULTS:

Sulfonylureas/Insulin vs. Dietary Therapy

- After treatment, the median HbA1c was 7.0% in the sulfonylurea/insulin group vs. 7.9% in the dietary group

- There were more hypoglycemic episodes in the sulfonylurea/insulin group than in the dietary group

- Patients in the sulfonylurea/insulin group gained an average of 2.9 kg more weight than those in the dietary group

Table 1: Summary of UKPDS's Key Findings[a]

Outcome	Sulfonylureas and Insulin Group (N=2,729)	Dietary Group (N=1,138)	P Value
Diabetes-related endpoints	40.9	46.0	0.03
Diabetes-related deaths	10.4	11.5	0.34
All-cause mortality	17.9	18.9	0.44
Microvascular disease	8.6	11.4	0.01

[a]Event rates are per 1000 person-years, i.e. the number of events that occurred for every 1000 years of participant time. For example, 40.9 events per 1000 person-years means that there were, on average, 40.9 events among 100 subjects who were each enrolled in the trial for ten years.

Metformin vs. Dietary Therapy and Sulfonylureas/Insulin (Overweight Patients)

- After treatment, the median HbA1c was 7.4% in the metformin group vs. 8.0% in the dietary group (patients in the sulfonylurea/insulin had similar HbA1c levels, as those in the metformin group, though the actual level was not reported)

- There were more hypoglycemic episodes among patients in the metformin group than among patients in the dietary therapy group, however patients in the insulin/sulfonylurea group had the highest rate of hypoglycemic episodes

- Patients in the metformin and dietary therapy groups had similar changes in body weight, while patients in the sulfonylurea/insulin group gained more weight than those in the metformin and dietary therapy groups

Table 2: UKPDS's Key Findings Among Overweight Patients[a]

Outcome	Metformin Group	Dietary Group	Sulfonylureas and Insulin Group	P Value[b]
	(N=342)	(N=411)	(N=951)	
Diabetes-related endpoints	29.8	43.8	40.1	0.0023, 0.0034
Diabetes-related deaths	7.5	12.7	10.3	0.017, non-significant[c]
All-cause mortality	13.5	20.6	18.9	0.011, 0.021
Microvascular disease	6.7	9.2	7.7	0.19, non-significant[c]

[a]Event rates are per 1000 person-years.
[b]Metformin vs. Dietary, Metformin vs. Sulfonylureas/Insulin
[c]Actual P-values not reported.

Criticisms and Limitations: UKPDS did not define appropriate HbA1c targets for patients with type 2 diabetes.

Other Relevant Studies and Information:

At the completion of the UKPDS trial, patients were managed for diabetes by their physicians. However, they continued to be monitored by the

UKPDS researchers for an additional 10 years. After a median of 16.8 years of follow-up in the sulfonylurea-insulin group and 17.7 years of follow-up in the metformin group, long term outcomes were reported[81]:

- Within a year of the trial's completion, average HbA1c levels were similar among all groups

- Patients in the sulfonylurea/insulin group still had fewer diabetes-related endpoints and less microvascular disease than those in the dietary group

- Patients in the sulfonylurea/insulin group had fewer myocardial infarctions and lower diabetes-related and all-cause mortality than those in the dietary group, findings that were not present in the initial analysis

- Overweight patients in the metformin group still had fewer diabetes-related endpoints, diabetes-related mortality, and all-cause mortality than those in the dietary group

The UKPDS trial also compared tight blood pressure control with an ACE inhibitor and beta-blocker (target blood pressure <150/85 mm Hg) vs. more lenient control (target blood pressure <180/105 mm Hg) among patients in the trial who had hypertension. Patients in the tight blood pressure control group had a reduction in total diabetes-related end points, diabetes-related death, stroke, and microvascular disease[82]. A follow-up analysis 10 years after the trial stopped did not demonstrate sustained benefits, however, suggesting that "good blood-pressure control must be continued if the benefits are to be maintained."[83]

The DCCT trial established the benefits of tight blood sugar control in preventing complications of type 1 diabetes[84].

81 Holman et al. 10-year follow-up of intensive glucose control in type 2 diabetes. N Engl J Med. 2008 Oct 9;359:2049-2056

82 UK Prospective Diabetes Study Group. Tight blood pressure control and risk of macrovascular and microvascular complications in type 2 diabetes: UKPDS 38. UK Prospective Diabetes Study Group. BMJ. 1998 Sep 12;317(7160):703-13.

83 Holman et al. Long-term follow-up after tight control of blood pressure in type 2 diabetes. N Engl J Med. 2008 Oct 9;359(15):1565-76.

84 The Diabetes Control and Complications Trial Research Group. The effect of intensive treatment of diabetes on the development and progression of long-term complications in insulin-dependent diabetes mellitus. N Engl J Med. 1993;329(14):977.

Other important studies examining glycemic control among patients with type 2 diabetes are described in the summary of the ACCORD trial.

SUMMARY AND IMPLICATIONS:

The UKPDS trial was the first study to conclusively show the benefits of medications for treating elevated blood sugar in patients with type 2 diabetes. Patients receiving sulfonylureas, insulin, and metformin had fewer diabetes-related complications than patient assigned to dietary therapy alone. The benefits of medications persisted 10 years after the trial was stopped.

CLINICAL CASE: TREATING ELEVATED BLOOD SUGAR LEVELS IN PATIENTS WITH TYPE 2 DIABETES

CASE HISTORY:

A 36 year old woman presents to your clinic with newly diagnosed type 2 diabetes. She is overweight with a body mass index of 36 kg/m^2 and does not exercise. Her HbA1c is 7.8%. Based on the results of the UKPDS trial, do you want to start this patient on medications to treat her elevated blood sugar?

SUGGESTED ANSWER:

The UKPDS trial was the first study to conclusively show the benefits of medications for treating elevated blood sugar in patients with type 2 diabetes. Patients receiving sulfonylureas, insulin, and metformin had fewer diabetes-related complications than patient assigned to dietary therapy alone.

The patient in this vignette is very young, however, and her HbA1c is only mildly elevated. While it would not be unreasonable to start her on a medication – probably metformin – an argument could also be made to encourage her to implement lifestyle changes first. If she were able to lose a considerable amount of weight and begin exercising, it is likely that her diabetes would improve and she might no longer require medications.

INTENSIVE VS. CONSERVATIVE BLOOD SUGAR CONTROL IN PATIENTS WITH TYPE 2 DIABETES:

THE "ACCORD" TRIAL[85]

"One message that has been pushed down our throats for over twenty years at least is that the lower your blood glucose levels are the better ... The surprising results of the [ACCORD trial are] that ... there were more deaths in the intensive therapy group than in the standard therapy group."

- Dr. David McCulloch
Clinical Professor of Medicine, University of Washington

---

85 Action to Control Cardiovascular Risk in Diabetes Study Group. Effects of intensive glucose lowering in type 2 diabetes. N Engl J Med. 2008 Jun 12;358(24):2545-59.

Research Question: Should doctors target a "normal" blood glucose level in patients with type 2 diabetes?

Funding: The National Heart, Lung, and Blood Institute (NHLBI)

Year Study Began: 2001

Year Study Published: 2008

Study Location: 77 centers in the U.S. and Canada

Who Was Studied: Patients 40-79 years old with type 2 diabetes, a hemoglobin A1C (HbA1c) ≥7.5%, and known cardiovascular disease or risk factors.

Who Was Excluded: Patients who were unwilling to do home blood glucose monitoring or unwilling to inject insulin; patients with frequent hypoglycemic episodes; and patients with a creatinine >1.5 mg/dl.

How Many Patients: 10,251

Study Overview:

Figure 1: Summary of ACCORD's Design

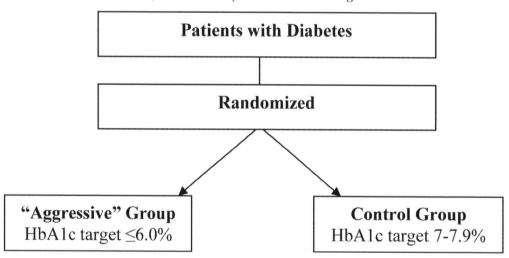

Study Intervention: Physicians could use any available diabetes medications to achieve the blood glucose targets. Metformin was used in 60% of the patients, insulin in 35%, and sulfonylureas in 50%.

Follow-Up: Mean of 3.5 years

Endpoints: Primary outcome: a composite of nonfatal myocardial infarction, nonfatal stroke, or death from cardiovascular causes. Secondary outcome: all-cause mortality.

RESULTS:

- the mean baseline HbA1c in both groups was 8.1%

- the mean post-treatment HbA1c in the "aggressive" group was 6.4% vs. 7.5% in the control group

- the mean weight gain in the "aggressive" group was 3.5 kg vs. 0.4 kg in the control group

Table 1: Summary of ACCORD's Key Findings

Outcome	"Aggressive" Group	Control Group	P Value
Hypoglycemia requiring medical assistance	10.5%	3.5%	<0.001
Cardiovascular events or cardiac death	6.9%	7.2%	0.16
All-cause mortality	5.0%	4.0%	0.04

Criticisms and Limitations: The study only included patients with cardiovascular disease or risk factors, and does not provide information about which medications may have been responsible for the excess mortality in the "aggressive group".

Other Relevant Studies and Information:

- The increased mortality rate among patients in the "aggressive" group persisted after five year follow-up[86].

- Another report involving the ACCORD data showed that, despite the increased mortality, patients in the "aggressive" group had lower rates of early-stage microvascular disease ("albuminuria and some eye complications and neuropathy")[87].

---

86 The ACCORD Study Group. Long-term effects of intensive glucose lowering on cardiovascular outcomes. N Engl J Med. 2011 Mar 3;364(9):818-28.

87 Ismail-Beigi et al. Effect of intensive treatment of hyperglycaemia on microvascular outcomes in type 2 diabetes: an analysis of the ACCORD randomised trial. Lancet. 2010 Aug 7;376(9739):419-30.

- The Veteran's Affairs Diabetes Trial (VADT) compared "aggressive" blood glucose management (targeting "normal" blood glucose levels) vs. standard glucose management and found no benefit of the aggressive approach[88].

- The ADVANCE trial found that patients treated for a HbA1c target of 6.5% had lower rates of diabetes-related complications, primarily nephropathy, than did patients treated for a standard HbA1c target[89].

- Most clinical practice guidelines recommend an HbA1c targets of 6.5-7.5%, and less aggressive targets for patients at high risk for hypoglycemia such as the elderly.

SUMMARY AND IMPLICATIONS:

A target HbA1c of ≤6.0% is associated with increased mortality compared with a target of 7.0%-7.9%.

CLINICAL CASE: INTENSIVE VS. CONSERVATIVE BLOOD SUGAR CONTROL

CASE HISTORY:

A 60 year old woman with long-standing type 2 diabetes, hypertension, and hyperlipidema presents for a routine office visit. Her diabetes medications include metformin 1000 mg twice daily, insulin glargine 40 units at bedtime, and regular insulin 12 units prior to each meal. She proudly shows you her blood sugar log, which demonstrates excellent sugar control with fasting morning sugars averaging 82. Her most recent HbA1c is 6.4%. Her only concerns are her continued inability to lose weight and occasional episodes of "shaking" when her blood sugars drop below 75.

After reading the ACCORD trial, what adjustments might you make to her diabetes medications?

---

88 Duckworth et al. Glucose Control and Vascular Complications in Veterans with Type 2 Diabetes. N Engl J Med. 2009 Jan 8;360(2):129-39.

89 The ADVANCE Collaborative Group. Intensive Blood Glucose Control and Vascular Outcomes in Patients with Type 2 Diabetes. N Engl J Med. 2008 Jun 12;358(24):2560-2572.

SUGGESTED ANSWER:

The ACCORD trial showed that aggressive blood sugar management with a target HbA1c of ≤6.0% was associated with increased mortality. In addition, targeting a HbA1c of ≤6.0% led to weight gain and an increased rate of hypoglycemic episodes. This patient's HbA1c is 6.4% – which was the mean HbA1c level in patients assigned to the "aggressive" blood sugar group in ACCORD. Thus, this patient's blood sugar control is probably too tight, and her insulin dose (either the insulin glargine, regular insulin, or both depending on her blood sugar patterns) should be reduced. This change would be expected to reduce the frequency of her hypoglycemic episodes, make it easier for her to lose weight, and perhaps reduce her risk of death.

THE AFRICAN AMERICAN HEART FAILURE TRIAL (A-HEFT)[90]

"Our finding of the efficacy of isosorbide dinitrate plus hy-dralazine in black patients provides strong evidence that this therapy can slow the progression of heart failure. A future strategy would be to identify genotypic and phenotypic characteristics that would transcend racial or ethnic categories to identify a population with heart failure in which there is an increased likelihood of a favorable response to such therapy."

- Taylor et al.[90]

Research Question: Is the combination of isosorbide dinitrate plus hydralazine effective for managing advanced heart failure in African Americans?

---

90 Taylor et al. Combination of isosorbide dinitrate and hydralazine in blacks with heart failure. N Engl J Med. 2004 Nov 11;351(20):2049-2056.

Funding: NitroMed Pharmaceuticals

Year Study Began: 2001

Year Study Published: 2004

Study Location: 161 centers in the U.S.

Who Was Studied: African Americans ≥18 with New York Heart Association class III or IV heart failure (patients with heart failure symptoms with minimal exertion or at rest). Patients were required to have a depressed ejection fracture (≤35% or <45% with a severely dilated left ventricle). In addition, patients were required to be on appropriate heart failure therapy (e.g. angiotensin-converting-enzyme inhibitors, beta-blockers, etc.).

The authors chose to study African Americans because retrospective studies had previously suggested that African Americans may respond particularly well to isosorbide dinitrate/hydralazine. In addition, African Americans have historically been under-represented in cardiovascular research.

Who Was Excluded: Patients with a recent cardiovascular event, clinically significant valvular disease, symptomatic hypotension, or another illness likely to result in death during the study period.

How Many Patients: 1,050

Study Overview:

Figure 1: Summary of A-HeFT's Design

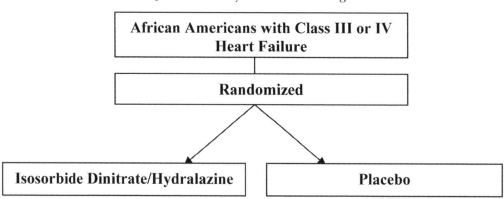

Study Intervention: Patients in the isosorbide dinitrate/hydralazine group initially received a tablet containing 20 mg of isosorbide dinitrate and 37.5 mg of hydralazine, which they were instructed to take three times daily. If tolerated, the dose was titrated up to two tablets three times daily. Patients in the placebo group received a placebo tablet that was administered according to the same protocol.

Follow-Up: Mean of 10 months

Endpoints: Primary outcome: a composite score incorporating death, a first hospitalization for heart failure, and change in the quality of life.

RESULTS:

- the trial was stopped early after it became clear that mortality rates were higher in the placebo group

- 47.5% of patients in the isosorbide dinitrate/hydralazine group reported headaches compared with 19.2% in the placebo group

- 29.3% of patients in the isosorbide dinitrate/hydralazine group reported dizziness compared with 12.3% in the placebo group

- the mean systolic blood pressure in the isosorbide dinitrate/hydralazine group dropped by 1.9 mm Hg, while the mean systolic blood pressure increased by 0.8 mm Hg in the placebo group

Table 2: Summary of A-HeFT's Key Findings

Outcome	Isosorbide Dinitrate/ Hydralazine Group	Placebo Group	P Value
Death	6.2%	10.2%	0.02
First hospitalization for heart failure	16.4%	24.4%	0.001
Change in quality of life[a]	-5.6	-2.7	0.02
Composite score[b]	-0.1	-0.5	0.01

[a]Quality of life was assessed using the "Minnesota Living with Heart Failure Questionnaire." A lower score indicates a higher quality of life, i.e. patients in the isosorbide dinitrate/hydralazine group reported a higher quality of life.
[b]A higher composite score indicates a better outcome, i.e. patients in the isosorbide dinitrate/hydralazine group had better outcomes.

Criticisms and Limitations: A-HeFT only included patients with advanced heart failure; whether isosorbide dinitrate/hydralazine is effective among patients with less severe disease is unclear.

Patients in the isosorbide dinitrate/hydralazine group experienced a considerably higher rate of headaches and dizziness compared to patients in the placebo group, highlighting the need to use the medications cautiously.

Other Relevant Studies and Information:

- The V-HeFT I trial showed that isosorbide dinitrate/hydralazine is superior to placebo among men with heart failure who were not taking angiotensin-converting-enzyme inhibitors[91].

- The V-HeFT II trial showed that the angiotensin-converting-enzyme inhibitor enalapril is superior to isosorbide dinitrate/hydralazine among men with heart failure[92].

SUMMARY AND IMPLICATIONS:

The A-HeFT trial showed that isosorbide dinitrate/hydralazine, when added to standard heart failure therapy, improves outcomes in African Americans with New York Heart Association class III or IV heart failure and a reduced ejection fraction. A-HeFT is also significant because it focused on African American patients who historically have been under-represented in medical research.

---

91 Cohn et al. Effect of vasodilator therapy on mortality in chronic congestive heart failure. Results of a Veterans Administration Cooperative Study. N Engl J Med. 1986;314(24):1547-52.

92 Cohn et al. A comparison of enalapril with hydralazine-isosorbide dinitrate in the treatment of chronic congestive heart failure. N Engl J Med. 1991;325(5):303-10.

CLINICAL CASE: ISOSORBIDE DINITRATE/ HYDRALAZINE FOR AFRICAN AMERICANS WITH HEART FAILURE

CASE HISTORY:

A 66 year old white man with New York Heart Association class IV heart failure (symptoms at rest) and an ejection fraction of 30% presents to your office for assistance in managing his symptoms. He reports taking lisinopril, carvedilol, spironolactone, amlodipine, furosemide, aspirin, atorvastatin, citalopram, gabapentin, and lorazepam. On exam, his HR is 72 and his blood pressure is 130/84. His lungs are clear and he has 1-2+ lower extremity edema.

Based on the results of A-HeFT, would you make any adjustments to this patient's medications to improve his heart failure therapy?

SUGGESTED ANSWER:

The A-HeFT trial demonstrated that isosorbide dinitrate/hydralazine, when added to standard heart failure therapy, improves outcomes in African Americans with New York Heart Association class III or IV heart failure and a reduced ejection fraction. Except for the fact that he is white, the patient in this vignette is typical of patients included in the trial. While one might argue that the results should not be applied to this patient because he is white, African American patients are frequently treated based on results of research that disproportionately involves white patients. For this reason, the author of this book believes that the results of A-HeFT should be applied to this patient, i.e. he should be a candidate for isosorbide dinitrate/ hydralazine.

On the other hand, however, the patient in this vignette is currently receiving 10 medications, and adding isosorbide dinitrate/hydralazine would further complicate his already complex medication regimen. Therefore, rather than adding isosorbide dinitrate/hydralazine, it might be preferable to increase the dose of another medication (perhaps the lisinopril) to help manage his symptoms. If isosorbide dinitrate/hydralazine is added, the patient should be monitored very carefully for hypotension and other side effects (headaches and dizziness).

EARLY VS. DELAYED ANTIRETROVIRAL THERAPY FOR PATIENTS WITH HIV:

THE NA-ACCORD STUDY[93]

"The results of this study suggest that among patients with a 351-500 CD4+ count, the deferral of antiretroviral therapy was associated with an increase in the risk of death of 69% ... Among patients with a more-than-500 CD4+ count, deferred therapy was associated with an increase in the risk of death of 94% ... [However] since patients in our study did not undergo randomization, the decision to initiate or defer antiretroviral therapy could have been influenced by multiple factors."

- Kitahata et al.[93]

93 Kitahata et al. Effect of early vs. deferred antiretroviral therapy for HIV on survival. N Engl J Med. 2009 Apr 30;360(18):1815-1826.

Research Question: At what CD4+ count should antiretroviral therapy be initiated in asymptomatic patients with HIV?

Funding: The National Institutes of Health and the Agency for Healthcare Research and Quality.

Year Study Began: data from 1996 – 2005 were included

Year Study Published: 2009

Study Location: data are from more than 60 sites in the U.S. and Canada

Who Was Studied: A cohort of asymptomatic U.S. and Canadian patients with HIV. Two separate analyses were performed, one involving patients with a CD4+ count of 351-500 cells per cubic millimeter and another in patients with a CD4+ count >500 cells per cubic millimeter.

Who Was Excluded: Patients with a previous AIDS-defining illness and those who had previously received antiretroviral therapy (ART).

How Many Patients: 17,517

Study Overview:

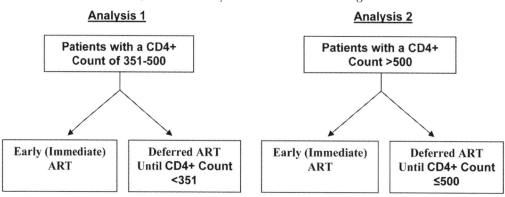

Figure 1: Summary of NA-ACCORD's Design

- Since this was not a randomized trial, patients chose whether they would receive early vs. deferred ART

- The authors adjusted the results for differences between patients in the early vs. deferred ART groups (e.g. for differences in baseline age and CD4+ count)

Study Intervention: In the first analysis, patients in the early therapy group received ART when their CD4+ counts were 351-500. Patient in the deferred therapy group did not receive ART until their counts were <351. Patients who initiated ART more than 6 months after having a measured CD4+ count of 351-500 but before their counts dropped below 351 were excluded.

In the second analysis, patients in the early therapy group received ART when their CD4+ counts were >500. Patient in the deferred therapy group did not receive ART until their counts were ≤500. Patients who initiated ART more than 6 months after having a measured CD4+ count of >500 but before their counts were ≤500 were excluded.

Follow-Up: Mean of 2.9 years

Endpoint: Death

RESULTS:

Analysis 1: CD4+ Count 351-500

- 8,362 patients were eligible for analysis 1, and of these patients 25% initiated early ART

- patients in the early therapy group were more likely to be white men and less likely to have a history of intravenous drug use and hepatitis C

Table 1: Summary of the Key Finding of Analysis 1

Outcome	Mortality Rate in Deferred ART Group[a]	Mortality Rate in Early ART Group[a]	Adjusted Odds Ratio for Deferred vs. Early ART	P Value
Death	5%	3%	1.69	<0.001

[a]Because of the complexity of these analyses, these rates are only approximates.

Analysis 2: CD4+ >500

- 9,155 patients were eligible for analysis 2, and of these patients 24% initiated early ART

- patients in the early therapy group were more likely to be white men and less likely to have a history of intravenous drug use and hepatitis C

- patients in the early therapy group had a higher rate of viral suppression after therapy initiation than patients in the deferred therapy group

(81% vs. 71%), suggesting better medication compliance in the early therapy group

Table 2: Summary of the Key Finding of Analysis 2

Outcome	Mortality Rate in Deferred ART Group[a]	Mortality Rate in Early ART Group[a]	Adjusted Odds Ratio for Deferred vs. Early ART	P Value
Death	5.1%	2.6%	1.94	<0.001

[a]Because of the complexity of these analyses, these rates are only approximates.

Criticisms and Limitations: The major limitation of NA-ACCORD is that it wasn't a randomized trial and even though the authors tried to adjust for differences between patients in the early vs. delayed therapy groups, it is possible that unmeasured confounding factors could have affected the results. For example, patients in the early therapy group may have been more engaged in their health than patients in the deferred therapy group, which may have led to improved survival among the early therapy patients. Indeed, patients in the early therapy group from analysis 2 had a higher rate of viral suppression than patients in the delayed ART group, suggesting a higher rate of medication compliance among early ART patients.

Another limitation of NA-ACCORD is that the authors did not report data on medication toxicity.

Other Relevant Studies and Information:

- High-quality randomized trials have convincingly demonstrated the benefit of ART in patients with a CD4+ count ≤200. In addition, strong evidence suggests that ART is beneficial in patients with CD4+ counts in the range of 200-350[94].

- Other studies besides NA-ACCORD have also suggested a benefit of ART in patients with CD4+ counts >350, most notably the SMART trial[95,96].

---

94 When to Start Consortium. Timing of initiation of antiretroviral therapy in AIDS-free HIV-1-infected patients: a collaborative analysis of 18 HIV cohort studies. Lancet. 2009;373(9672):1352.

95 SMART Study Group. CD4+ count-guided interruption of antiretroviral treatment. N Engl J Med. 2006;355(22):2283.

96 SMART Study Group. Major clinical outcomes in antiretroviral therapy (ART)-naive participants and in those not receiving ART at baseline in the SMART study. J Infect Dis. 2008;197(8):1133.

- Most guidelines recommend the initiation of ART for asymptomatic patients with CD4+ counts under 500[97] as well as in selected patients with CD4+ counts ≥500 (such as patients with a history of opportunistic infections and those with certain direct complications of HIV such as HIV nephropathy).

- A number of randomized trials are underway to more definitively determine the optimal strategy for initiating ART in asymptomatic patients.

SUMMARY AND IMPLICATIONS:

Although NA-ACCORD was not a randomized trial and therefore the conclusions are far from definitive, the results suggest that initiation of ART in self-selected asymptomatic patients with HIV is beneficial when the CD4+ count is 351-500 as well as when the count is >500.

CLINICAL CASE: EARLY VS. DELAYED ANTIRETROVIRAL THERAPY FOR PATIENTS WITH HIV

CASE HISTORY:

A 34 year old man with a history of intravenous drug use presents to your HIV clinic for a follow-up evaluation. He has missed three out of his last four clinic appointments, and admits to continued intermittent IV drug use. His most recent CD4+ count, measured two months ago, was 542 and his viral load was 36,000 copies/ml. The patient asks you if he should start taking medications to treat his HIV.

Based on the results of NA-ACCORD, how should you respond?

SUGGESTED ANSWER:

NA-ACCORD suggests that initiation of ART in asymptomatic patients with HIV and a CD4+ count >500 is beneficial. However, since NA-ACCORD was not a randomized trial, the results are not definitive. Most guidelines

---

97 Thompson et al. Antiretroviral treatment of adult HIV infection: 2010 recommendations of the International AIDS Society-USA panel. JAMA. 2010;304(3):321.

only recommend the initiation of ART for a selected group of asymptomatic patients with CD4+ counts ≥500 (such as patients with a history of opportunistic infections and those with certain direct complications of HIV such as HIV nephropathy). Not only does this patient not meet any of these criteria, but he also has exhibited behavior that raises questions about his ability to comply with ART. Rather than initiate ART, you should educate the patient about the need to take better care of himself (i.e. to stop using IV drugs). In addition, since he likely will require ART in the near future, you should educate him about the importance of medication adherence.

EARLY VS. LATE INITIATION OF DIALYSIS:

THE IDEAL TRIAL[98]

"[With] careful clinical management of chronic kidney disease, dialysis can be delayed for some patients until the [glomerular filtration rate] drops below 7.0 ml per minute or until more traditional clinical indicators for the initiation of dialysis are present."

- Cooper et al.[98]

Research Question: Can the initiation of dialysis safely be delayed in patients with an estimated glomerular filtration rate (GFR) ≤14.0 ml per minute who do not demonstrate traditional signs or symptoms indicating the need for dialysis?

Funding: The trial was supported by grants from several public research agencies in Australia and New Zealand, three pharmaceutical and/or medical device companies, and by the non-profit International Society for Peritoneal Dialysis.

Year Study Began: 2000

98 Cooper et al. A randomized, controlled trial of early vs. late initiation of dialysis. N Engl J Med. 2010 Aug 12;363(7):609-619.

Year Study Published: 2010

Study Location: 32 centers in Australia and New Zealand

Who Was Studied: Patients ≥18 with progressive chronic kidney disease and an estimated GFR between 10.0 - 15.0 ml per minute per 1.73 m² of body-surface area (determined using the Cockcroft-Gault equation[99] and corrected for body-surface area). Patients with kidney transplants were included in the study.

Who Was Excluded: Patients with a GFR <10.0 ml per minute, those with plans to receive a live-donor kidney transplant within the next 12 months, and those with a recently diagnosed cancer likely to impact survival.

How Many Patients: 828

Study Overview:

Figure 1: Summary of IDEAL's Design

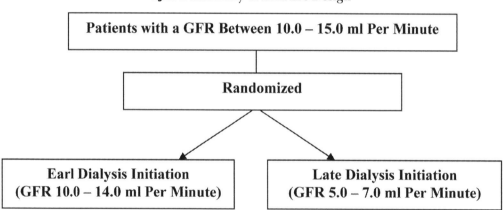

Study Intervention: Patients assigned to the early dialysis group began dialysis when their GFR was between 10.0 – 14.0 ml per minute while those assigned to the late dialysis group began dialysis when their GFR was between 5.0 – 7.0 ml per minute. Patients in the late start group could also initiate dialysis when their GFR was >7.0 ml per minute at their physicians' discretion (e.g. due to symptoms of uremia or difficult-to-manage electrolyte disturbances).

Patients and their physicians selected the method of dialysis (i.e. peritoneal dialysis vs. hemodialysis) and the dialysis regimen in both groups.

Follow-Up: A median of 3.59 years

---

99 Cockcroft DW and Gault MH. Prediction of creatinine clearance from serum creatinine. Nephron 1976;16:31-41.

Endpoints: Primary outcome: All-cause mortality. Secondary outcomes: cardiovascular events (e.g. myocardial infarctions, strokes, or hospitalizations for angina); infectious events (deaths or hospitalizations due to an infection); complications of dialysis (e.g. temporary placement of an access catheter or fluid or electrolyte disorders); and quality of life.

RESULTS:

- the mean age of study patients was approximately 60 years

- the most common cause of renal failure among study patients was diabetes (approximately 34%)

- 98% of patients who survived until the end of the trial ultimately required dialysis

- the median time until dialysis initiation in the early start group was 1.80 months vs. 7.40 months in the late start group (P<0.001) and the mean estimated GFR at dialysis initiation was 12.0 ml per minute in the early start group vs. 9.8 ml per minute in the late start group (P<0.001)

- 75.9% of patients in the late start group initiated dialysis before their GFR dropped below 7.0 due to signs or symptoms indicating the need for dialysis

Table 1: Summary of IDEAL's Key Findings[a]

Outcome	Early Dialysis Group	Late Dialysis Group	P Value
Death from Any Cause	10.2	9.8	0.75
Cardiovascular Events	10.9	8.8	0.09
Infectious Events	12.4	14.3	0.20
Complications of Dialysis			
Temporary catheter placement	10.0	9.7	0.85
Access-site infection	3.4	3.5	0.97
Fluid or electrolyte disorder	13.2	15.0	0.26

[a]Event rates are per 100 patient-years, i.e. the number of events that occurred for every 100 years of patient time. For example, 10.2 deaths per 100 patient-years means that, on average, 10.2 patients died for every 25 patients who were each enrolled in the trial for four years.

- quality of life scores (as measured by the Assessment of Quality of Life instrument[100]) were similar between the early and late start groups

Criticisms and Limitations: Although early dialysis initiation provided no apparent benefit, most patients in the late initiation group required dialysis during the study period before reaching a GFR of 5.0 – 7.0 ml per minute.

Other Relevant Studies and Information:

- An economic analysis of data from IDEAL demonstrated that dialysis costs were significantly higher in the early initiation group and total costs were non-significantly higher[101]

- Guidelines from the National Kidney Foundation, published before the results of IDEAL were available, suggest that dialysis should be considered in patients with a GFR <15 ml per minute[102]

- Among patients who initiated dialysis in the U.S. in 2005, 45% had an estimated GFR >10.0 ml per minute – more than double the rate in 1996[103]

SUMMARY AND IMPLICATIONS:

With appropriate clinical management, patients with progressive chronic kidney disease can safely delay dialysis initiation until they either develop signs or symptoms indicating the need for dialysis or until their GFR drops below 7.0 ml per minute. Although most patients in the late start group required dialysis before their GFR dropped below 7.0, patients were able to delay dialysis initiation by an average of 6 months without any adverse effects.

---

100 Hawthorne et al. The assessment of quality of life (AQoL) instrument: a psychometric measure of health-related quality of life. Qual Life Res 1999;8:209-24.

101 Harris et al. Cost-effectiveness of initiating dialysis early: a randomized controlled trial. Am J Kidney Dis. 2011 May;57(5):707-15.

102 K/DOQI Clinical Practice Guidelines and Clinical Practice Recommendations 2006 Updates Hemodialysis adequacy Peritoneal Dialysis Adequacy Vascular Access. Am J Kidney Dis. 2006; 48(Suppl 1):S1.

103 Rosansky et al. Initiation of dialysis at higher GFRs: is the apparent rising tide of early dialysis harmful or helpful? Kidney Int 2009;76:257-61.

CLINICAL CASE: EARLY VS. LATE INITIATION OF DIALYSIS

CASE HISTORY:

A 56 year old woman with chronic kidney disease due to diabetes presents for an initial evaluation in the nephrology clinic at an urban medical center. The patient was referred for nephrology consultation almost two years ago, however there is a long back-log for nephrology appointments and the nephrologists are overwhelmed with patients. The woman is currently asymptomatic, and her estimated GFR is 12. Her physical examination is normal, as are her electrolytes.

As a nephrologist in this clinic, and based on the results of the IDEAL trial, do you feel comfortable delaying dialysis initiation in this patient until she develops a "hard" indication such as a difficult-to-manage electrolyte disturbance?

SUGGESTED ANSWER:

The IDEAL trial demonstrated that, with appropriate monitoring, patients with progressive chronic kidney disease can safely delay dialysis initiation until they either develop signs or symptoms indicating the need for dialysis or until their GFR drops below 7.0 ml per minute. Thus, under ideal circumstances, the patient in this vignette would be able to delay dialysis initiation.

This patient receives care at an under-resourced medical center, however, and the nephrology staff may not be able to monitor her closely over the next several months. Without appropriate monitoring, this patient is at risk for a life-threatening complication. Thus, given the resource limitations, it might be appropriate to initiate dialysis immediately.

EARLY GOAL-DIRECTED THERAPY
IN SEPSIS[104]

"[Goal-directed therapy aimed at restoring] a balance between oxygen delivery and oxygen demand ... [in] the earliest stages of severe sepsis and septic shock ... has significant short-term and long-term benefits."

- Rivers et al.[104]

Research Question: Does aggressive correction of hemodynamic disturbances in the early stages of sepsis improve outcomes?

Funding: Henry Ford Health Systems Fund for Research and a Weatherby Healthcare Resuscitation Fellowship.

Year Study Began: 1997

Year Study Published: 2001

Study Location: The Henry Ford Hospital in Detroit, Michigan

---

104 Rivers et al. Early goal-directed therapy in the treatment of severe sepsis and septic shock. N Engl J Med. 2001 Nov 8;345(19):1368-77.

Who Was Studied: Adults presenting to the emergency room with severe sepsis or septic shock. To qualify, patients needed to have a suspected infection and at least two of four criteria for a systemic inflammatory response syndrome (SIRS) as well as a systolic blood pressure ≤90 mm Hg. Alternatively, they could have a suspected infection, at least two SIRS criteria, and a lactate ≥4.0 mm/L.

Table 1: SIRS Criteria

Temperature	≤36° C or ≥38° C
Heart rate	≥90
Respiratory rate	≥20 or $PaCO_2$ <32 mm Hg
White cell count	≥12,000 or ≤4,000 or ≥10% bands

Who Was Excluded: Patients who were pregnant, as well as those with several acute conditions including: stroke, acute coronary syndrome, acute pulmonary edema, status asthmaticus, or gastrointestinal bleeding. In addition, patients with a contraindication to central venous catheterization were excluded.

How Many Patients: 263

Study Overview:

Figure 1: Summary of the Trial Design

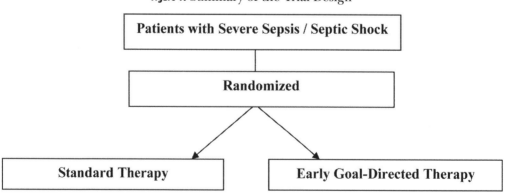

Study Intervention: Patients in the standard therapy group received immediate critical care consultation and were admitted to the intensive care unit as quickly as possible. Subsequent management was at the discretion of the critical care team, which was given a protocol advocating the following hemodynamic goals:

- 500-ml boluses of crystalloid should be given every 30 minutes as needed to achieve a central venous pressure (CVP) of 8-12 mm Hg

- vasopressors should be used as needed to maintain a mean arterial pressure (MAP) ≥65 mm Hg

- urine output goal ≥0.5 ml/kg/hr

Patients in the early goal-directed therapy group were managed according to a similar protocol, however they also received central venous oxygen saturation (ScvO$_2$) monitoring from a specialized central line catheter:

- if the ScvO$_2$ was <70%, red cells were transfused to achieve a hematocrit ≥30%

- if the transfusion was ineffective, dobutamine was given as tolerated

In addition, and perhaps most importantly, patients in the early goal-directed therapy group received six hours of aggressive treatment *immediately* upon presentation to the emergency room.

Follow-Up: 60 days

Endpoints: Primary outcome: in-hospital mortality.

RESULTS:

- during the first six hours, patients in the early goal-directed therapy group received more fluid, more blood transfusions, and more inotropic support than did patients in the standard therapy group

- during the first six hours, patients in the early goal-directed group had higher average MAPs, and a higher average ScvO$_2$; in addition, a higher proportion achieved the combined goals for CVP, MAP, and urine output

- during the period from 7-72 hours, patients in the early goal-directed therapy group had better hemodynamic parameters, and required less fluid, red cell transfusions, vasopressors, and mechanical ventilation

Table 2: Summary of the Trial's Key Findings

Outcome	Standard Therapy Group	Early Goal-Directed Therapy Group	P Value
Hospital length of stay[a]	18.4 days	14.6 days	0.04
60-day mortality	56.9%	44.3%	0.03
In-hospital mortality	46.5%	30.5%	0.009

[a]Among patients who survived to hospital discharge.

Criticisms and Limitations: The early goal-directed protocol involved several interventions, and therefore it is not possible to know which of these measures were most important for improving outcomes. In particular, some experts have questioned the importance of aggressive red cell transfusions and dobutamine administration based on $ScvO_2$ measurements.

Other Relevant Studies and Information: A recent trial comparing hemodynamic monitoring with $ScvO_2$ measurements vs. lactate clearance in patients with sepsis suggested that the two forms of monitoring are equivalent[105].

SUMMARY AND IMPLICATIONS:

Most patients with severe sepsis or septic shock should be managed with aggressive hemodynamic monitoring and support immediately upon presentation in the emergency room (or, if this is not possible, in the intensive care unit) for 6 hours or until there is resolution of hemodynamic disturbances.

CLINICAL CASE: EARLY GOAL-DIRECTED THERAPY

CASE HISTORY:

A 48 year old previously healthy man presents reporting that he "feels miserable." Over the past day, he has had a cough with thick green sputum as well as subjective fevers and fatigue. The symptoms worsened two hours prior to presentation, and he now has rigors, increasing fatigue, and mild

---

105 Jones et al. Lactate clearance vs central venous oxygen saturation as goals of early sepsis therapy: a randomized clinical trial. JAMA. 2010 Feb 24;303(8):739-46.

to moderate dyspnea. On exam, his temperature is 39° C, his heart rate is 126, his respiratory rate is 24, and his blood pressure is 96 mm Hg / 64 mm Hg. His labs are notable for a white blood cell count of 18,000 with 40% bands and a lactate of 3.0 mm/L. His chest x-ray shows a right middle lobe consolidation.

After reading this trial about early goal directed therapy, how would you treat this patient upon presentation to the emergency room?

SUGGESTED ANSWER:

This patient fulfills more than two SIRS criteria and has a suspected infection (pneumonia). However, he doesn't quite fulfill the criteria for severe sepsis specified in the trial since his systolic blood pressure is >90 mm Hg and his lactate is <4.0 mm/L. If he did meet the criteria for severe sepsis, he should be treated immediately (in the emergency room if possible) with early goal directed therapy:

- 500-ml boluses of crystalloid every 30 minutes for a target CVP of 8-12 mm Hg

- vasopressors to maintain a MAP ≥65 mm Hg

- urine output goal ≥0.5 ml/kg/hr

- hemodynamic monitoring with $ScvO_2$ measurements (or lactate clearance measurements) and red cell transfusions followed by cautious dobutamine administration to achieve the hemodynamic goals

Even though this patient does not quite fulfill the criteria for severe sepsis, it might still be reasonable to implement early goal directed therapy because he is so close to meeting the criteria. At the very least, he should be closely monitored and early goal directed therapy instituted immediately if his systolic blood pressure were to drop below 90 mm Hg or his lactate were to drop below 4.0 mm/L.

RED CELL TRANSFUSION IN CRITICALLY ILL PATIENTS:

THE TRICC TRIAL[106]

"Our findings indicate that the use of a threshold for red-cell transfusion as low as 7.0 [grams] of hemoglobin per deciliter … was at least as effective as and possibly superior to a liberal transfusion [threshold of 10.0 g/dl] in critically ill patients …"

- Hébert et al.[106]

Research Question: When should patients in the intensive care unit (ICU) with anemia receive red cell transfusions?

Funding: The Medical Research Council of Canada and an unrestricted grant from the Bayer company (the Bayer grant was given after funding had been secured from the Medical Research Council of Canada).

Year Study Began: 1994

---

106 Hébert et al. A multicenter, randomized, controlled clinical trial of transfusion requirements in critical care. N Engl J Med. 1999 Feb 11;340(6):409-17.

Year Study Published: 1999

Study Location: 25 intensive care units in Canada

Who Was Studied: Adults in medical and surgical intensive care units with a hemoglobin (hgb) <9.0 g/dl, and who were clinically euvolemic.

Who Was Excluded: Patients with considerable active blood loss (e.g. gastrointestinal bleeding leading to a drop in hgb of at least 3.0 points in the preceding 12 hours), chronic anemia (documented hgb <9.0 g/dl at least one month before admission), and those who were pregnant.

How Many Patients: 838

Study Overview:

Figure 1: Summary of TRICC's Design

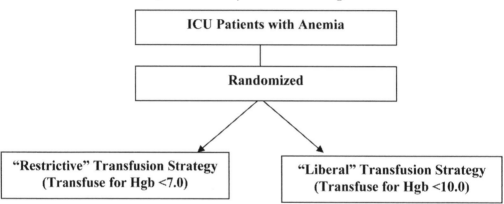

Study Intervention: Non-leukoreduced red cells were transfused according to the above thresholds and were given one unit at a time. After each transfusion, the patient's hemoglobin was measured and additional transfusions were given as needed.

Follow-Up: 30 days

Endpoints: Primary outcome: 30-day mortality. Secondary outcomes: 60-day mortality, multi-organ failure.

RESULTS:

- approximately 30% of patients had a primary respiratory diagnosis; 20% had a primary cardiac diagnosis; 15% had a primary gastrointestinal illness; and for 20%, the primary diagnosis was trauma

- patients in the "restrictive" group received an average of 2.6 units of blood during the trial, compared to an average of 5.6 units in the liberal group

- the average daily hgb in the "restrictive" group was 8.5 vs. 10.7 in the "liberal" group

Table 1: Summary of TRICC's Key Findings

Outcome	"Restrictive" Group	"Liberal" Group	P Value
30-day mortality	18.7%	23.3%	0.11
60-day mortality	22.7%	26.5%	0.23
Multi-organ failure[a]	5.3%	4.3%	0.36

[a]More than three failing organs.

- as indicated in Table 1, there was no significant difference in 30-day mortality between patients in the "restrictive" vs. "liberal" groups, however in a subgroup analysis involving younger and healthier patients 30-day mortality rates were significantly lower in the "restrictive" group

- in another subgroup analysis involving patients with cardiac disease, there was no significant difference in 30-day mortality between patients in the "restrictive" vs. "liberal" groups, however patients with acute coronary syndromes had non-significantly improved outcomes with the "liberal" transfusion strategy[107]

- cardiac events (pulmonary edema and myocardial infarction) were significantly more common in the "liberal" group

Criticisms and Limitations: A disproportionate number of patients with severe cardiac disease did not participate in the trial because their physicians chose

---

107 Hébert et al. Is a low transfusion threshold safe in critically ill patients with cardiovascular diseases? Crit Care Med. 2001;29(2):227.

not to enroll them. In addition, the red cells used in this trial were not leukocyte-reduced. Some centers now routinely use leukocyte-reduced blood, which may be associated with few transfusion-related complications.

Other Relevant Studies and Information:

- A review of trials comparing restrictive vs. liberal transfusion strategies concluded that "existing evidence supports the use of restrictive transfusion [strategies] in patients who are free of serious cardiac disease", however "the effects of conservative transfusion [strategies] on functional status, morbidity and mortality, particularly in patients with cardiac disease, need to be tested in further large clinical trials."[108]

- Trials have supported the use of a restrictive transfusion strategy in patients undergoing elective coronary artery bypass surgery[109], patients who have undergone surgery for a hip fracture[110], and children in the intensive care unit[111]

- A small trial involving elderly patients admitted to the hospital with a hip fracture compared a liberal transfusion strategy (hgb threshold ≤10 g/dl) vs. a restrictive strategy (hgb threshold ≤8 g/dl). The trial showed lower mortality with the liberal strategy, however these findings require replication in a larger study[112].

SUMMARY AND IMPLICATIONS:

For most critically ill patients, waiting to transfuse red cells until the hgb drops below 7.0 is at least as effective as, and likely preferable to, transfusing at a hgb less than 10.0. These findings may not apply to patients with acute blood loss or chronic anemia who were excluded from the trial. The results also may not apply to patients with active cardiac ischemia who were poorly

---

108 Carless et al. Transfusion thresholds and other strategies for guiding allogeneic red blood cell transfusion. Cochrane Database Syst Rev. 2010 Oct 6;(10):CD002042.

109 Bracey et al. Lowering the hemoglobin threshold for transfusion in coronary artery bypass procedures: effect on patient outcome. Transfusion. 1999;39(10):1070.

110 Carson et al. Liberal or restrictive transfusion in high-risk patients after hip surgery. NEJM. 2011;365(26:2453.

111 Lacroix et al. Transfusion strategies for patients in pediatric intensive care units. N Engl J Med. 2007 Apr 19;356(16):1609-19.

112 Foss et al. The effects of liberal vs. restrictive transfusion thresholds on ambulation after hip fracture surgery. Transfusion. 2009;49(2):227.

represented in the trial and had non-significantly worse outcomes with a transfusion threshold of 7.0.

CLINICAL CASE: RED CELL TRANSFUSION IN CRITICALLY ILL PATIENTS

CASE HISTORY:

A 74 year old woman with myelodysplastic syndrome is admitted to the general medicine service at your hospital with pneumonia. On review of systems, you note that she has suffered from increasing fatigue for the past 3 months. Her hgb on admission is 8.0 g/dl – which has decreased from 10.5 g/dl when it was last measured 4 months ago.

Based on the results of the TRICC trial, should you give this patient a red cell transfusion?

SUGGESTED ANSWER:

The TRICC trial showed that, for most critically ill patients, waiting to transfuse red cells until the hgb drops below 7.0 g/dl is at least as effective as, and likely preferable to, transfusing at a hgb <10.0 g/dl. However, the patient in this vignette is not critically ill, and thus the results of TRICC should not be applied to her. This patient's fatigue likely results from anemia due to her myelodysplastic syndrome. Red cell transfusion would likely be appropriate for her.

PULMONARY ARTERY CATHETERS IN CRITICALLY ILL PATIENTS[113]

"[C]linical management involving early use of a [pulmonary artery catheter] was not associated with significant changes in mortality and morbidity among patients with shock, [acute respiratory distress syndrome], or both."

- Richard et al.[113]

Research Question: Do critically ill patients benefit from early insertion of a pulmonary artery catheter to help guide management?

Funding: Two French governmental agencies and a company that manufactures medical devices.

Year Study Began: 1999

Year Study Published: 2003

Study Location: 36 intensive care units in France

113 Richard et al. Early use of the pulmonary artery catheter and outcomes in patients with shock and acute respiratory distress syndrome. JAMA. 2003 Nov 26;290(20):2713-2720.

Who Was Studied: Patients with shock, acute respiratory distress syndrome (ARDS), or both.

Who Was Excluded: Patients with hemorrhagic shock, those with a myocardial infarction complicated by cardiogenic shock and requiring revascularization, and those with a platelet count ≤10,000 per microliter. In addition, patients meeting criteria for shock for over 12 hours were excluded.

How Many Patients: 676

Study Overview:

Figure 1: Summary of the Trial's Design

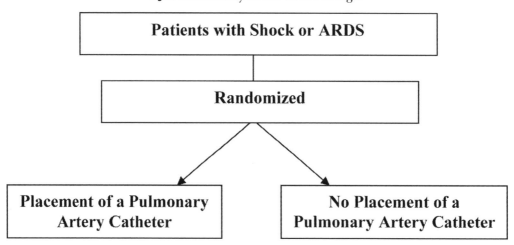

Study Intervention: Patients assigned to the pulmonary artery catheter group received a catheter within two hours of enrollment. The type of catheter was determined by the care team as was the site of catheter insertion. Additionally, the decision about when to remove the catheter or whether to replace it was left to the care team. The care team could use data from the catheter to guide therapy (e.g. physicians could adjust medications based on the pressure readings), however the care team was not given specific protocols to follow.

Patients in the control group did not receive a catheter but otherwise received standard care.

Follow-Up: 28 days

Endpoints: Primary outcome: Mortality after 28 days. Secondary outcomes: Length of stay in the hospital and intensive care unit (ICU), organ system failure, and the need for mechanical ventilation, dialysis, or vasoactive medications.

RESULTS:

- In the control group, a pulmonary artery catheter was inserted in 4.4% of patients despite the fact that this violated the study protocol

- In the catheter group, 2.4% of patients did not receive a catheter (six died before catheter insertion while in two catheter placement was not possible)

- In patients in the catheter group, the catheter remained in place for a mean of 2.3 days

- During catheter insertion, approximately 5% of patients experienced an arterial puncture and approximately 18% experienced arrhythmias or conduction disturbances; there were no deaths directly attributable to catheter insertion, however

Table 1: Summary of the Trial's Key Findings

Outcome	Pulmonary Artery Catheter Group	Control Group	P Value
28 Day Mortality	59.4%	61.0%	0.67
ICU Length of Stay	11.6 days	11.9 days	0.72
Hospital Length of Stay	14.0 days	14.4 days	0.67

- There were no significant differences between patients in the pulmonary artery catheter group vs. patients in the control group with respect to organ system failure or the need for mechanical ventilation, dialysis, or vasoactive medications

Criticisms and Limitations: The study was underpowered for detecting small differences in outcomes between patients in the catheter vs. control groups.

Physicians treating patients in the catheter group used data from the pulmonary artery catheters to guide therapy, however they were not given specific protocols to follow. It is possible that catheterization might have resulted in a significant benefit if the care teams had been given management protocols.

Other Relevant Studies and Information:

- A number of other randomized trials in critically ill patients have also failed to show a benefit of pulmonary artery catheterization[114,115].

- A trial of pulmonary artery catheterization in patients admitted to the hospital for heart failure did not demonstrate a benefit[116], nor did a trial of pulmonary artery catheterization in high-risk patients prior to surgery[117].

- Because of these findings, pulmonary artery catheters are used much less commonly now than in the past.

SUMMARY AND IMPLICATIONS:

In critically ill patients, pulmonary artery catheterization did not lead to improved outcomes compared to standard care without catheterization. This trial, along with other trials of pulmonary artery catheterization, demonstrates the importance of evaluating widely used technologies that have never been adequately assessed.

CLINICAL CASE: PULMONARY ARTERY CATHETERS IN CRITICALLY ILL PATIENTS

CASE HISTORY:

A 60 year old man was admitted to the intensive care unit 36 hours ago with severe pancreatitis. He was intubated on admission due to tachypnea and hypoxemia. He continues to have a high oxygen requirement with a PaO_2 of 95 mm Hg despite receiving an FiO_2 of 0.60. His chest x-ray shows

---

114 Shah et al. Impact of the pulmonary artery catheter in critically ill patients: meta-analysis of randomized clinical trials. JAMA. 2005;294(13):1664.

115 National Heart, Lung, and Blood Institute Acute Respiratory Distress Syndrome (ARDS) Clinical Trials Network. Pulmonary-artery vs. central venous catheter to guide treatment of acute lung injury. N Engl J Med. 2006;354(21):2213.

116 Binanay et al. Evaluation study of congestive heart failure and pulmonary artery catheterization effectiveness: the ESCAPE trial. JAMA. 2005;294(13):1625.

117 Sandham et al. A randomized, controlled trial of the use of pulmonary-artery catheters in high-risk surgical patients. N Engl J Med. 2003;348(1):5.

bilateral pulmonary infiltrates, and an echocardiogram shows no evidence of cardiac dysfunction.

The attending pulmonologist would like to place a pulmonary artery catheter to help guide management. She says, "How else am I supposed to know whether the patient needs more diuresis?"

Based on the results of this trial of pulmonary artery catheterization, do you agree with the pulmonologist's recommendation?

SUGGESTED ANSWER:

Existing data, including this trial, do not suggest that pulmonary artery catheterization in critically ill patients is beneficial. In addition, pulmonary artery catheterization may lead to complications (according to this trial, the risk of arterial puncture is approximately 5% while the risk of arrhythmias or conduction disturbances is approximately 18%). Therefore, pulmonary artery catheterization is generally not indicated for patients like the one in this vignette.

STEP-UP VS. STEP-DOWN THERAPY FOR DYSPEPSIA:

THE DIAMOND TRIAL[118]

"[For patients with new onset dyspepsia] a step-up strategy starting with antacids is more cost effective than a step-down strategy starting with proton pump inhibitors ... [The two approaches have] equal clinical effectiveness ... at 6 months ..."

- van Marrewijk et al.[118]

Research Question: Which is more effective for the management of new onset dyspepsia: a step-up strategy in which patients are first given an antacid, followed by an H_2-receptor antagonist, and then a proton pump inhibitor, or a step-down strategy in which a proton pump inhibitor is given first, followed by an H_2-receptor antagonist, and then an antacid? Also, which of these strategies is more cost effective?

---

118 van Marrewijk et al. Effect and cost-effectiveness of step-up vs. step-down treatment with antacids, H_2-receptor antagonists, and proton pump inhibitors in patients with new onset dyspepsia (DIAMOND study): a primary-care-based randomized controlled trial. The Lancet. 2009 Jan 17;373:215-225.

Funding: The Netherlands Organization for Health Research and Development.

Year Study Began: 2003

Year Study Published: 2009

Study Location: 312 Dutch family doctors participated

Who Was Studied: Patients ≥18 years old presenting to their primary physician with new onset dyspepsia. Patients with reflux-predominant dyspepsia were included.

Who Was Excluded: Patients who had a upper endoscopy in the previous year, those who had used acid-suppressive medications in the previous 3 months, and those with alarm symptoms (dysphagia, unintended weight loss, anemia, or hematemesis).

How Many Patients: 664

Study Overview:

Figure 1: Summary of DIAMOND's Design

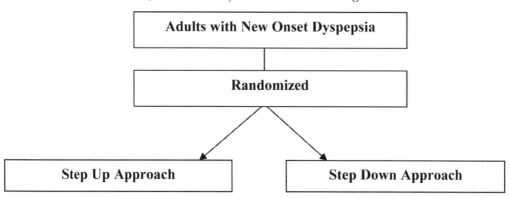

Study Intervention: Patients assigned to the step-up therapy group received medications in the following sequence:

- antacid therapy (aluminum oxide 200 mg/magnesium hydroxide 400 mg four times daily)

- H_2-receptor antagonist (ranitidine 150 mg twice daily)

- proton pump inhibitor (pantoprazole 40 mg once daily)

Patients assigned to the step-down therapy group received medications in the following sequence:

- proton pump inhibitor (pantoprazole 40 mg once daily)

- H$_2$-receptor antagonist (ranitidine 150 mg twice daily)

- antacid therapy (aluminum oxide 200 mg/magnesium hydroxide 400 mg four times daily)

In both groups, patients were treated with each medication for four weeks. If the first medication in the sequence had insufficient effect, patients were given the second medication. If the second medication had insufficient effect, they were given the third medication. When any of these medications was successful, therapy was stopped, however If the symptoms relapsed within 4 weeks, medications were resumed at the next step in the sequence (e.g. in the step-down group, if a proton pump inhibitor was successful but the patient relapsed within 4 weeks, an H$_2$-receptor antagonist was started). In both groups, when none of the three medications was effective, or for relapses after 4 weeks, patients were managed according to usual practice by their physicians.

Patients in both groups were otherwise evaluated and counseled by their physicians according to standard practice. Diagnostic testing (e.g. *H. pylori* testing and endoscopy) prior to and during treatment was left to the discretion of the treating physician.

Follow-Up: 6 months

Endpoints: Primary outcomes: adequate symptom relief and cost-effectiveness. Secondary outcomes: gastrointestinal symptom severity, quality of life, and absenteeism from work.

Symptom relief was assessed by asking patients whether their symptoms were adequately relieved.

The costs of each treatment strategy were estimated by adding the costs of medications (including medications given outside of the study protocol), physician visits (for both primary and specialty care), and diagnostic tests (e.g. *H. pylori* testing, endoscopies, and abdominal imaging) in each group. In addition, costs from decreased productivity were estimated based on patient reports and added to the total.

RESULTS:

- in the step-up group, 100% of patients received antacids, 59% received an H_2-receptor antagonist, and 35% received a proton pump inhibitor

- in the step-down group, 100% of patients received a proton pump inhibitor, 53% received an H_2-receptor antagonist, and 35% received antacids

- there were no significant differences in the number of primary care or specialty physician visits, diagnostic testing (*H. pylori* testing, endoscopy, or abdominal imaging), or absenteeism from work between the groups

Table 1: DIAMOND's Key Findings

Outcome	Step-Up Group	Step-Down Group	P Value
Adequate symptom relief at 4 weeks	55%	66%	Significant[a]
Adequate symptom relief at 6 months	72%	70%	0.63
Mean costs per patient[b,c]	€426	€460	0.02

[a]Exact P-value not reported.
[b]Cost reported in euros.
[c]When cost calculations were performed using generic medication costs, rather than brand medication costs, the cost difference between the groups was no longer significant.

Criticisms and Limitations: Many physicians follow different empiric medication protocols than those used in this trial. For example, many physicians would not prescribe an H_2-receptor antagonist or an antacid to patients who did not respond to a proton pump inhibitor. In addition, patients who respond to a dyspepsia medication but relapse shortly after stopping it would commonly be restarted on the same effective medication rather than being switched to another medication.

Only a small percentage of patients in this study had reflux-predominant symptoms. Other studies have suggested that these patients may respond better to proton pump inhibitors.

In the cost analysis, the step-up approach was not significantly more cost effective than the step-down approach when generic medication costs, rather than brand name medication costs, were used.

Other Relevant Studies and Information:

- The American Gastroenterological Association recommends that patients with new onset dyspepsia be tested for *H. pylori* and treated if positive. For patients negative for *H. pylori,* as well as those with persistent symptoms after *H. pylori* therapy, the guidelines recommend empiric proton pump inhibitors.

SUMMARY AND IMPLICATIONS:

For patients with new-onset dyspepsia, a step-up strategy in which patients are first given an antacid, followed by an H_2-receptor antagonist, and then a proton pump inhibitor was as effective as a step-down strategy in which a proton pump inhibitor is given first, followed by an H_2-receptor antagonist, and then an antacid (though symptom relief occurred slightly more quickly with a step-down approach). The step-up strategy was more cost effective. Since the protocols used in this study were different from those frequently used in practice, these results do not definitively show that a step-up approach is preferable. Still, despite expert guidelines to the contrary, the DIAMOND trial shows that a step-up approach is a reasonable strategy for treating dyspepsia.

CLINICAL CASE: STEP-UP VS. STEP-DOWN THERAPY FOR DYSPEPSIA

CASE HISTORY:

A 32 year old man presents with vague epigastric discomfort. The symptoms have been present intermittently for the past few years, and frequently get worse after meals. The man denies alarm symptoms (dysphagia, unintended weight loss, anemia, or hematemesis), and his physical examination is normal.

Based on the results of DIAMOND, how should you treat this patient?

SUGGESTED ANSWER:

The DIAMOND trial showed that a step-up strategy for managing dyspepsia is as effective as a step-down strategy, though symptom relief occurred slightly more quickly with a step-down approach. The step-up strategy was more cost effective.

The patient in this vignette presents with dyspepsia. Based on recommendations from the American Gastroenterological Association, you might consider testing this patient for *H. pylori* and treating him if positive. Assuming that the *H. pylori* test is negative – or that the symptoms persist after treatment for *H. pylori* – you could initiate empiric therapy. Since step-up therapy was found to be more cost-effective in DIAMOND, you might opt to start with an antacid such as aluminum oxide/magnesium hydroxide. Regardless of whether you opt for a step-up vs. a step-down approach, however, it will be important to monitor the patient closely (including an evaluation of the patient's compliance with treatment) and adjust therapy based on his response.

OPIOIDS FOR CHRONIC NON-CANCER PAIN[119]

"[Among patients with non-cancer-related chronic pain] and in whom there is no history of substance abuse ... nine weeks of oral morphine ... may be of analgesic benefit, but is unlikely to confer psychological or functional improvement ... Further randomized controlled trials are required to define the role of oral morphine in the management of chronic non-cancer pain."

- Moulin et al.[119]

Research Question: Do patients with chronic pain not due to cancer benefit from treatment with opioids?

Funding: The Medical Research Council of Canada and Purdue Frederick, a pharmaceutical company that manufactures opioids.

Year Study Began: Mid 1990's

---

119 Moulin et al. Randomised trial of oral morphine for chronic non-cancer pain. Lancet. 1996;347:143-147.

Year Study Published: 1996

Study Location: A pain clinic at Victoria Hospital in Ontario, Canada

Who Was Studied: Adults 18-70 with stable non-cancer-related pain of ≥6 months duration and of at least moderate intensity (≥5 on a 1-10 scale). Patients were required to have "regional pain of a myofascial, musculoskeletal, or rheumatic nature." In addition, all study patients had failed to respond to non-steroidal anti-inflammatory drugs and at least one month of tricyclic antidepressant therapy.

Who Was Excluded: Patients with a history of substance abuse, those with a history of psychosis or a major mood disorder, those with neuropathic pain syndromes such as reflex sympathetic dystrophy, those with isolated headache syndromes (since opioids may lead to rebound headaches), and those with other medical problems such as congestive heart failure that might complicate opioid therapy. In addition, patients were excluded if they had previously received opioids for chronic pain (prior codeine treatment was allowed since codeine is available over-the-counter in Canada).

How Many Patients: 61

Study Overview:

Figure 1: Summary of the Trial's Design

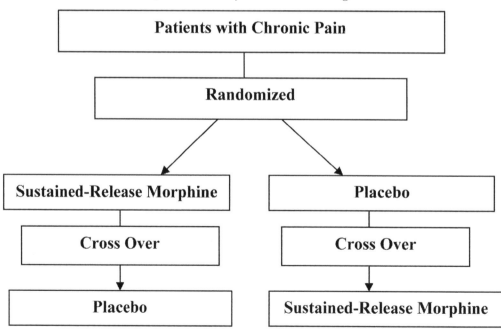

Study Intervention: Patients assigned to the morphine group received sustained-release morphine (MS Contin). The medication was titrated over three weeks, initially at a dose of 15 mg twice daily up to a maximum of 60 mg twice daily if tolerated. The medication was then continued at the maximum tolerated dose for an additional six weeks before being tapered over two weeks.

Patients assigned to the placebo group received benztropine – a medication with "no analgesic properties" but that "mimics many of the possible side-effects of morphine." The benztropine was titrated in a similar fashion, initially at a dose of 0.25 mg twice daily up to a maximum of 1.0 mg twice daily if tolerated. Benztropine was then continued at the maximum tolerated dose for an additional six weeks before being tapered over two weeks.

At the completion of the taper, patients in both groups crossed over and received 11 weeks of the other therapy (i.e. all patients ultimately received 11 weeks of morphine and 11 weeks of placebo).

Patients in both groups could take paracetamol (acetaminophen) as a "rescue medication" when necessary. In addition, all study patients were offered group sessions led by a psychologist to learn "cognitive-behavioral strategies for pain management" (patients were not required to participate in these sessions).

Follow-Up: 11 weeks

Endpoints: Primary outcome: Patient-reported pain intensity on a 1-10 scale (1=lowest intensity, 10=highest intensity). Secondary outcomes: Use of paracetamol for breakthrough pain; and scores on a panel of questionnaires measuring psychological and functional improvement.

RESULTS:

- the mean age of study patients was 40, and the mean duration of pain symptoms was 4.1 years

- 25% of the patients were employed, 85% had injury-related pain, and 41% had previously consulted ≥5 specialists about their pain

- 38% of patients primarily suffered from head, neck, and shoulder pain while 34% primarily suffered from back pain

- the mean total daily dose of morphine tolerated by study patients was 83.5 mg

Table 1: Pain Intensity Scores (Scale 1-10)[a]

Group	Baseline	9 Weeks[b]	11 Weeks[c]	P Value[d]
Morphine	7.8	7.1	7.3	0.01
Placebo	7.8	7.9	8.5	

[a]These data are only from the first phase of the study prior to the cross over. Similar findings were noted when data from the second phase (after the cross over) were included.
[b]At the completion of full-dose treatment.
[c]At the completion of the washout period.
[d]Comparison is for change in pain scores during phase 1 of the study in the morphine vs. placebo groups.

Table 2: Other Outcomes

Outcome	Morphine Group	Placebo Group	P Value
Tabs of Paracetamol Required Per Day for Breakthrough Pain	3.5	3.9	0.40
Psychological Well-Being[a]	67.7	67.7	Not Significant[b]
Quality of Life			
Sickness Impact Profile[c]	24.5	24.2	Not Significant[b]
Pain Disability Index[d]	44.6	45.0	Not Significant[b]

[a]As assessed by the Symptom Check List-90, which is scored based on patient responses to a questionnaire from 30 to 81 "with higher scores indicating greater impairment."
[b]Actual p values not reported.
[c]Scored based on patient responses to a questionnaire on a scale of 0-100 with "higher values indicating worse function."
[d]Scored based on patient responses to a questionnaire on a scale of 0-70 with "higher values indicating worse function."

- there appeared to be a "carryover effect" in which patients who received morphine during the first phase of the study had lower pain intensity scores during the second phase after being switched to placebo (the authors hypothesize that this may have been due to a persisting "psychological effect" from morphine)

- patients in the morphine group were more likely than patients in the placebo group to experience vomiting (43% vs. 6%, P=0.0002), dizziness (50% vs. 15%, P=0.0004), constipation (56% vs. 19%, P=0.0005), and abdominal pain (29% vs. 11%, P=0.04)

- 8.7% of patients in the morphine group vs. 4.3% in the placebo group reported drug craving (difference not significant)

- 41.3% of patients preferred treatment with morphine, 28.3% preferred treatment with placebo, and 30.4% had no preference (P=0.26)

Criticisms and Limitations: The patients were only followed for 11 weeks and thus this study did not assess the long term impact of opioid therapy.

Patients in this study were monitored very closely (they had visits with the study team every 1-2 weeks). It is uncertain whether opioid therapy would have the same effects in a less closely monitored setting more typical of a "real-world" environment.

Patients with substance abuse disorders were excluded from the study and thus the results do not apply to these patients.

Other Relevant Studies and Information:

- There have been surprisingly few other studies evaluating the use of opioids for the treatment of chronic non-cancer pain. Most other studies were also small, had a follow-up of <16 weeks, and compared opioids with placebo (rather than with another active therapy). These studies have generally come to similar conclusions as this study, namely that opioids lead to a modest reduction in pain scores and, at best, a small improvement in functional outcomes[120,121]

- Opioids are widely felt to be appropriate for chronic use in patients with pain due to cancer and other life-threatening conditions, and many experts believe that opioids are under-prescribed among these patients

- Opioids have become one of the most widely used medications in the U.S.[122]

- Guidelines from the American Pain Society state that "although evidence is limited ... chronic opioid therapy can be an effective therapy for carefully selected and monitored patients with chronic non-cancer pain. However, opioids are also associated with potentially serious

---

120 Kalso et al. Opioids in chronic non-cancer pain: systematic review of efficacy and safety. Pain. 2004 Dec;112(3):372-80.

121 Furlan et al. Opioids for chronic noncaner pain: a meta-analysis of effectiveness and side effects. CMAJ. 2006;174(11):1589-1594.

122 Okie S. A flood of opioids, a rising tide of deaths. NEJM. 2011;364(4):290.

harms, including opioid-related adverse effects and outcomes related to the abuse potential of opioids."[123]

SUMMARY AND IMPLICATIONS:

Among patients with non-cancer related pain, sustained-release oral morphine led to a modest reduction in pain but no clear improvement in psychological or functional outcomes. Patients in the morphine group experienced an increased rate of gastrointestinal symptoms and dizziness. The study had important methodological limitations, most notably that patients were only followed for 11 weeks. In addition, patients with a history of substance abuse were excluded, limiting the generalizability of the findings. Despite these limitations, this study represents one of the highest quality studies to evaluate opioids for chronic non-cancer pain.

CLINICAL CASE: OPIOIDS FOR NON-CANCER PAIN

CASE HISTORY:

A 28 year old woman presents to your clinic after returning from combat in Afghanistan with chronic neck pain. Her symptoms began after a whiplash injury suffered during combat. The pain has persisted for almost a year, and substantially interferes with her life. She reports difficulty sleeping due to the pain, and says that the pain reaches at least 7 on a scale from 1-10 most days of the week. She has tried over-the-counter pain medications, including acetaminophen and ibuprofen, however these medications "barely take the edge off."

The patient tells you that her friend was recently given morphine and Vicodin (acetaminophen and hydrocodone) for back pain, and this seems to have helped. The patient wonders whether she might benefit from these medications as well. What can you tell her based on the results of this study?

SUGGESTED ANSWER:

This patient has chronic, non-cancer related pain that substantially interferes with her life. Studies evaluating opioids for chronic non-cancer related pain

---

123 American Pain Society. Guideline for the use of opioid therapy in chronic noncancer pain: evidence review. Glenview, IL: American Pain Society; 2009.

indicate that these medications may reduce pain in the short term. However, data on outcomes after 16 weeks are scant, and the impact of opioids on psychological and functional outcomes are uncertain. In addition, opioids lead to significant side-effects and potentially addiction in some high risk patients. For these reasons, non-opioid treatment options should be fully explored before starting chronic opioid therapy.

The patient in this vignette has tried over-the-counter pain medications, but should also try non-pharmacological strategies for pain management such as physical therapy or cognitive-behavioral therapy. If these strategies prove ineffective, you might consider a long-acting medication for chronic pain such as amitriptyline. In the meantime, the patient could continue using non-narcotic pain relievers such as acetaminophen and ibuprofen. It would also be reasonable to prescribe a small supply of a short-acting opioid medication such as an acetaminophen and hydrocodone combination (Vicodin) for episodes of severe pain. (The patient might use this medication when she has difficulty sleeping.)

If non-opioid therapy is ultimately ineffective, it would be appropriate to consider opioid therapy (others might reasonably decide not to use opioids in a patient such as this, however). If the decision to initiate opioids is made, it would first be necessary to evaluate risk factors for substance abuse. In addition, the patient should agree to a pain contract stating that opioids are only to be prescribed by one provider (usually the primary care provider or a pain specialist) as well as other stipulations to ensure safe use.

SECTION 3:

SURGERY

PERIOPERATIVE BETA-BLOCKERS IN NON-CARDIAC SURGERY:

THE POISE TRIAL[124]

"[Although perioperative metoprolol] reduced the risk of myocardial infarction ... compared with placebo, the drug also resulted in a significant excess risk of death, stroke, and clinically significant hypotension and bradycardia."

- POISE Study Group[124]

Research Question: Should patients undergoing non-cardiac surgery receive a perioperative beta-blocker to prevent cardiovascular complications?

---

124 POISE Study Group. Effects of extended-release metoprolol succinate in patients undergoing non-cardiac surgery (POISE trial): a randomised controlled trial. Lancet. 2008 May 31;371(9627):1839-47.

Funding: Governmental agencies from Canada, Australia, Spain, and Great Britain. AstraZeneca also provided a small portion of the funding.

Year Study Began: 2002

Year Study Published: 2008

Who Was Studied: Adults ≥45 undergoing non-cardiac surgery with an expected hospital length of stay ≥24 hours and who had or were at risk for atherosclerotic disease. Patients undergoing elective, urgent, and emergent surgeries were all included.

Who Was Excluded: Patients with a heart rate <50, those with a second or third degree heart block, and those with asthma (since beta-blockers can trigger asthma exacerbations). In addition, patients were excluded if they were already receiving a beta-blocker or verapamil, had a known history of an adverse reaction to beta-blockers, or were undergoing a "low-risk surgical procedure (based on the individual physician's judgment)."

How Many Patients: 8,351

Study Overview:

Figure 1: Summary of POISE's Design

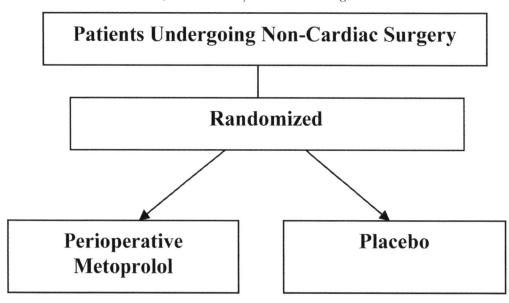

Study Intervention: Patients assigned to the metoprolol group received oral extended-release metoprolol starting 2-4 hours before surgery. Patients had their blood pressure and heart rate measured prior to medication administration and the dose was held in patients with a heart rate <50 or a systolic blood pressure <100 mm Hg. Patients also received postoperative extended-release metoprolol as follows:

- at any point in the first six hours following surgery, patients received a dose of metoprolol 100 mg if the heart rate was ≥80 and the systolic blood pressure ≥100 mm Hg

- patients who did not receive metoprolol within the first six hours received a 100 mg dose six hours after surgery

- 12 hours after the first postoperative dose, patients began taking metoprolol 200 mg daily for 30 days

- metoprolol was held and the dose was reduced to 100 mg once daily in patients who had a heart rate <50 or a systolic blood pressure <100 mm Hg

Patients who could not take oral medications received intravenous metoprolol until they were able to tolerate oral medications.

Patients assigned to the placebo group were treated with placebo according to the same schedule.

Follow-Up: 30 days

Endpoints: Primary outcome: a composite of cardiovascular death, non-fatal myocardial infarction, and non-fatal cardiac arrest at 30 days. Secondary outcomes: clinically significant hypotension, clinically significant bradycardia, stroke, and death.

RESULTS:

- data from 752 patients were excluded due to fraudulent activity and data from 8351 patients were analyzed in the final analysis

- the mean age of study subjects was 69, the mean preoperative heart rate was 78, and the mean preoperative blood pressure was 139 mm Hg / 78 mm Hg

- 42% of patients underwent vascular surgery, 22% intraperitoneal surgery, and 21% orthopedic surgery

Table 1: Summary of POISE's Key Findings

Outcome	Metoprolol Group	Placebo Group	P Value
Cardiovascular Death, Myocardial Infarction, and Cardiac Arrest	5.8%	6.9%	0.039
Non-fatal Myocardial Infarction[a]	3.6%	5.1%	0.0008
Clinically Significant Hypotension	15.0%	9.7%	<0.0001
Clinically Significant Bradycardia	6.6%	2.4%	<0.0001
Stroke	1.0%	0.5%	0.0053
Death	3.1%	2.3%	0.0317

[a]Two thirds of the myocardial infarctions did not result in ischemic symptoms. Myocardial infarctions in these patients were diagnosed based on elevations of cardiac biomarkers and an additional defining feature of myocardial infarction (e.g. ischemic ECG changes or wall motion abnormalities on an echocardiogram).

Criticisms and Limitations: It is possible that the results would have been different if a different beta-blocker or different dose had been used, or if the medication had been given according to a different dosing schedule.

Other Relevant Studies and Information:

- A meta-analysis of over 30 trials evaluating the use of peri-operative beta-blockers was consistent with POISE[125]

- Small trials using low dose beta-blockers[126] and in which the beta-blocker was initiated at least a week prior to surgery[127] have suggested a benefit of perioperative beta blockade in preventing cardiovascular complications, however there were methodological limitations to these studies and the reliability of the results of one of these studies has been called into qustion[127]

---

125 Bangalore et al. Perioperative beta blockers in patients having non-cardiac surgery: a meta-analysis. Lancet. 2008;372(9654):1962.

126 Mangano et al. Effect of atenolol on mortality and cardiovascular morbidity after non-cardiac surgery. NEJM. 1996; 335:1713-20.

127 Poldermans et al. The effect of bisoprolol on perioperative mortality and myocardial infarction in high-risk patients undergoing vascular surgery. NEJM. 1999; 341:1789-94.

- Guidelines published after POISE emphasize that evidence supporting initiation of perioperative beta blockade is weak. When beta-blockers are initiated perioperatively – something which is not necessarily recommended – they should only be given to high risk patients undergoing intermediate to high risk surgeries, and should be started at low doses (target heart rate 60-80) at least a week beforehand. Patients already receiving beta-blockers should be continued on them perioperatively, however, since rapid withdrawal of beta-blockers may lead to cardiovascular complications[128].

SUMMARY AND IMPLICATIONS:

The initiation of perioperative extended-release metoprolol in patients not currently taking a beta-blocker lowers the risk of myocardial infarction but leads to clinically significant bradycardia and hypotension, and increases the risk of stroke and overall mortality. It is possible that, when initiated at least several days prior to surgery and at appropriate doses, some high risk patients may benefit from the initiation of perioperative beta-blockers. However, existing evidence does not provide support for the initiation of perioperative beta-blockers in most patients not currently taking these medications.

CLINICAL CASE: PERIOPERATIVE BETA BLOCKADE

CASE HISTORY:

A 70 year old woman is brought to the emergency department by ambulance after a bystander found her clutching her abdomen on the street. The patient is in severe pain and tells you she has "heart problems" but cannot recall her medications. Her heart rate is 110 and her blood pressure is 160 mm Hg / 100 mm Hg. A CT scan of her abdomen shows evidence of an acute intra-abdominal process and she is scheduled for an urgent laparotomy.

Based on the results of POISE, should you treat this patient with a perioperative beta-blocker?

---

128 American College of Cardiology Foundation/American Heart Association Task Force on Practice Guidelines. 2009 ACCF/AHA focused update on perioperative beta blockade. J Am Coll Cardiol. 2009;54(22):2102.

SUGGESTED ANSWER:

The POISE trial does not support the routine initiation of perioperative beta-blockers in patients undergoing non-cardiac surgery. However, patients chronically receiving beta-blockers were excluded from POISE since rapid withdrawal of beta-blockers may lead to cardiovascular complications.

We do not know whether the patient in this vignette regularly receives a beta-blocker. If she does, the beta-blocker should be continued as long as her heart rate and blood pressure can tolerate it. But if she doesn't, a beta-blocker probably should not be started.

Given the uncertainty, common sense should be used in managing this patient. Because she has cardiovascular disease and her heart rate and blood pressure are elevated, it might be reasonable to cautiously initiate a low dose, short acting beta-blocker and monitor her carefully for brady-cardia and hypotension. However, it would be equally correct to withhold a beta-blocker, particularly post-operatively since monitoring on surgical floors is often sparse.

CARDIAC STENTS VS. CORONARY ARTERY BYPASS SURGERY FOR SEVERE CORONARY ARTERY DISEASE:

THE SYNTAX TRIAL[129]

"[Patients with three-vessel and/or left main coronary artery disease] treated with [percutaneous coronary intervention] involving drug-eluting stents were more likely than those undergoing [coronary artery bypass grafting] to reach the primary end point of the study – death from any cause, stroke, myocardial infarction, or repeat revascularization ... [However, patients undergoing stenting] were less likely to have a stroke."

- Lange and Hillis[130]

---

129 Serruys et al. Percutaneous coronary intervention vs. coronary-artery bypass grafting for severe coronary artery disease. N Engl J Med. 2009 Mar 5;360(10):961-972.

130 Lange RA and Hillis LD. Coronary revascularization in context. N Engl J Med. 2009;360:1024-1026.

Research Question: Should patients with severe coronary artery disease (three-vessel and/or left main disease) be treated with percutaneous coronary intervention (PCI) or coronary artery bypass grafting (CABG)?

Funding: Boston Scientific, which manufactures cardiac stents.

Year Study Began: 2005

Year Study Published: 2009

Study Location: 85 sites in 17 countries in the U.S. and Europe

Who Was Studied: Patients with ≥50% stenosis in at least three coronary arteries or in the left main coronary artery in whom "equivalent anatomical revascularization could be achieved with either CABG or PCI" as judged by a cardiologist and cardiac surgeon. Patients were also required to have symptoms of stable or unstable angina, atypical chest pain, or, if asymptomatic, evidence of myocardial ischemia on a stress test.

Who Was Excluded: Patients with prior PCI or CABG, those with an acute myocardial infarction (MI), and those requiring another cardiac surgery.

How Many Patients: 1,800

Study Overview:

Figure 1: Summary of the Trial's Design

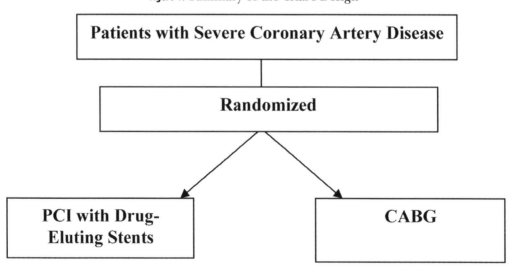

Study Intervention: Patients assigned to both the PCI and CABG groups underwent the procedures according to local practice. Patients in the PCI group received drug-eluting stents. The goal of therapy in both groups was

complete revascularization of all target vessels. Adjunctive peri-procedural and post-procedural therapy, including anti-platelet therapy, was also provided according to local practice.

Follow-Up: 12 months

Endpoints: Primary outcome: A composite of major cardiovascular and cerebrovascular events (death from any cause, stroke, MI, or repeat revascularization). Each component of this composite was also assessed individually.

RESULTS:

- the mean age of study participants was 65, approximately 25% had diabetes, 57% had stable angina, 28% had unstable angina, and 2% had an ejection fraction <30%

- patients in the PCI group received an average of >4 stents each

- patients in the PCI had a shorter length of hospital stay (3.4 days vs. 9.5 days, P<0.001)

- patients in the PCI received more aggressive post-procedure medication therapy (e.g. more patients received antiplatelet medications, warfarin, statins, and ACE inhibitors), however more patients in the CABG group received amiodarone

Table 1: Summary of SYNTAX's Key Findings

Outcome	PCI Group	CABG Group	P Value
Major Cardiovascular or Cerebrovascular Events	17.8%	12.4%	0.002
Death	4.4%	3.5%	0.37
Stroke	0.6%	2.2%	0.003
Myocardial Infarction	4.8%	3.3%	0.11
Repeat Revascularization	13.5%	5.9%	<0.001

- the authors also report stratified patient outcomes using a prediction rule – called the SYNTAX score – that classifies coronary artery disease by its complexity (e.g. patients with coronary lesions that are anatomically more difficult to access with PCI receive a higher score); the SYNTAX score may help predict which patients are good candidates for PCI

Criticisms and Limitations: If patients in the CABG group had received post-procedure medication therapy similar to that received by patients in the PCI group, the benefits of CABG vs. PCI may have been more pronounced.

Other Relevant Studies and Information:

- A follow-up analysis of data from the SYNTAX trial reported that 76.3% of patients in the CABG group vs. 71.6% of patients in the PCI group were free from symptoms of angina after 12 months (P=0.05)[131].

- Additional follow-up data from SYNTAX were presented at the European Association of Cardio-Thoracic Surgery 2011 Annual Meeting. After 4 years of follow-up, patients in the CABG group were reported to have lower rates of all-cause morality, cardiac mortality, and myocardial infarction compared with patients in the PCI group.

- Trials prior to the advent of drug-eluting stents that compared PCI with CABG in patients with multi-vessel disease demonstrated similar results as SYNTAX[132].

- The STICH trial, which compared coronary-artery bypass surgery vs. medical therapy in patients with coronary artery disease and an ejection fraction ≤35%, found that the two treatments led to similar mortality rates[133].

SUMMARY AND IMPLICATIONS:

For patients with three-vessel and/or left main coronary artery disease, CABG reduced rates of major cardiovascular and cerebrovascular events compared with PCI. This difference was largely driven by a reduction in the need for repeat revascularization procedures among patients receiving CABG. Patients who received PCI had a lower rate of stroke,

---

131 Cohen et al. Quality of life after PCI with drug-eluting stents or coronary artery bypass surgery. N Engl J Med. 2011 Mar 17;364:1016-1026.

132 Daemen et al. Long-term safety and efficacy of percutaneous coronary intervention with stenting and coronary artery bypass surgery for multivessel coronary artery disease: a meta-analysis with 5-year patient-level data from the ARTS, ERACI-II, MASS-II, and SoS trials. Circulation 2008;118:1146-54.

133 Velazquez et al. Coronary-artery bypass surgery in patients with left ventricular dysfunction. NEJM. 2011;364:1607-16.

however, which may make PCI an attractive option for some patients. In addition, the authors suggest that patients with less complex coronary artery disease (as assessed using the SYNTAX score) may be particularly good candidates for PCI, but this hypothesis requires further validation.

CLINICAL CASE: REVASCULARIZATION AMONG PATIENTS WITH SEVERE CORONARY ARTERY DISEASE

CASE HISTORY:

An 86 year old man visits his doctor because of increasing shortness of breath when walking. The symptoms have been getting progressively worse over the past month. At baseline, the patient could walk for three blocks without resting, and now he can barely walk for one block. A cardiac stress test with nuclear imaging demonstrates reversible ischemia in the territory of the left main coronary artery.

Based on the results of the SYNTAX trial, do you believe that this patient should be treated with PCI or with CABG?

SUGGESTED ANSWER:

SYNTAX showed that, for patients with three-vessel and/or left main coronary artery disease, CABG lowered rates of major cardiovascular and cerebrovascular events compared with PCI. However, patients in the CABG group experienced a higher rate of stroke.

The patient in this vignette is much older than the typical patient in SYNTAX (approximately 65). Because of his advanced age and limited performance status, the less invasive treatment – PCI – would likely be preferable for him. In addition, he would be less likely to experience a stroke – which could be a devastating complication for him at this stage in his life. This case highlights why, despite the fact that CABG proved superior to PCI in SYNTAX, some patients may still reasonably opt for PCI.

CAROTID ENDARTERECTOMY FOR ASYMPTOMATIC CAROTID STENOSIS:

THE ACST TRIAL[134,135]

"Among [asymptomatic] patients ... with severe carotid stenosis ... [carotid endarterectomy] approximately halved the net 5-year risk of stroke ... [however] the balance of risk and benefit depends on surgical morbidity rates ... and on the risk of carotid stroke in the absence of surgery."

- The ACST Collaborative Group[134]

134 Halliday et al. MRC Asymptomatic Carotid Surgery Trial Collaborative Group. Prevention of disabling and fatal strokes by successful carotid endarterectomy in patients without recent neurological symptoms: randomized controlled trial. Lancet. 2004 May 8;363(9420):1491-502.

135 Halliday et al. 10-year stroke prevention after successful carotid endarterectomy for asymptomatic stenosis (ACST-1): a multicentre randomised trial. Lancet. 2010 Sep 25;376(9746):1074-84.

Research Question: Is carotid endarterectomy (CEA) beneficial in asymptomatic patients with severe carotid stenosis?

Funding: The United Kingdom Medical Research Council and the Stroke Association.

Year Study Began: 1993

Year Study Published: 2004

Study Location: 126 hospitals in 30 countries

Who Was Studied: Asymptomatic adults 40-91 years old with unilateral or bilateral carotid artery stenosis of at least 60% on ultrasound.

Who Was Excluded: Patients with a stroke, transient cerebral ischemia, or other relevant neurological symptoms in the past six months; patients with a prior ipsilateral CEA; patients at high surgical risk; and patients with other major medical problems. In addition, surgeons with high complication rates (>6% rates of perioperative stroke or death) were not eligible to participate in the trial.

How Many Patients: 3,120

Study Overview:

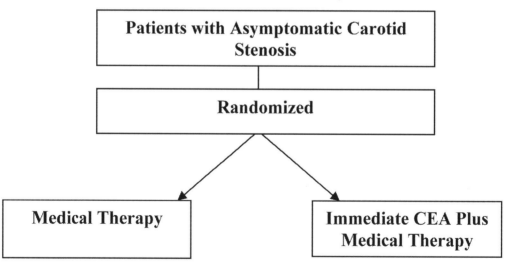

Figure 1: Summary of ACST's Design

Study Intervention: Patients in the CEA group were offered the procedure immediately. In contrast, patients in the medical therapy group only received surgery if they developed symptoms due to the stenosis, if a "hard" indication for CEA arose, or if "the doctor or patient changed their mind". In both groups, patients received standard medical care for atherosclerotic disease with antiplatelet agents, blood pressure medications, and lipid-lowering therapy.

Follow-Up: Mean of 7 years

Endpoints: Perioperative mortality, perioperative stroke, and non-operative stroke.

RESULTS:

- approximately 90% of patients in the CEA group underwent CEA within a year of enrollment vs. approximately 5% of patients in the medical therapy group (typically due to the development of a "hard" indication for CEA)

- approximately 26% of patients in the medical therapy group underwent CEA within 10 years of enrollment (again, typically due to the development of a "hard" indication for CEA)

- 2.8% of patients in the CEA group experienced perioperative stroke or death

- for the first two years of the trial, patients in the medical therapy group had better outcomes than those in the CEA group because of the high rate of perioperative strokes and death among patients assigned to CEA, however after two years, the benefits of CEA became apparent as shown in Table 1

Table 1: ACST's Key Findings[a]

Outcome	Medical Therapy Group	CEA Group	P Value
Stroke or perioperative death	17.9%	13.4%	0.009
Non-perioperative stroke	16.9%	10.8%	0.0004

[a]Projected 10-year cumulative event rates

- Both men and women ultimately benefited from CEA, however patients >75 at trial entry did not

Criticisms and Limitations: Since the time ACST was conducted, medical therapy for atherosclerotic disease has improved. For example, at the beginning of the trial, just 17% of patients were taking lipid-lowering medications. It is possible that the benefits of CEA may be less pronounced now that medical therapies have improved. However, in ACST both patients who were receiving lipid-lowering therapy as well as those who weren't did benefit from CEA.

In addition, surgeons with high complication rates were not invited to participate in the trial, and therefore it is possible that the benefits of CEA may be lower in "real world setting" in which some CEAs are performed by less skilled surgeons. However, the 3% perioperative complication rates reported in ACST are similar to complication rates reported in large European registries.

Other Relevant Studies and Information:

- Two other large trials, a VA study[136] and the ACAS trial[137], also evaluated CEA in asymptomatic patients and came to similar conclusions as the ACST trial.

- A meta-analysis involving data from ACAS and ACST raised questions about the effectiveness of CEA for asymptomatic carotid disease among women[138]. This meta-analysis did not include long term follow-up data from ACST, however, and the benefits of CEA in women take longer to become apparent.

- Studies have also demonstrated the benefit of CEA in patients with symptomatic carotid disease, most notably the NASCET[139] and ECST[140] trials.

---

136 Hobson et al. Efficacy of carotid endarterectomy for asymptomatic carotid stenosis. N Engl J Med 1993 Jan 28;328(4):221-7.

137 Executive Committee for the Asymptomatic Carotid Atherosclerosis Study. Endarterectomy for asymptomatic carotid artery stenosis. JAMA 1995 May 10;273(18):1421-8.

138 Rothwell et al. Carotid endarterectomy for asymptomatic carotid stenosis: asymptomatic carotid surgery trial. Stroke 2004; 35:2425

139 North American Symptomatic Carotid Endarterectomy Trial Collaborators. Beneficial effect of carotid endarterectomy in symptomatic patients with high-grade carotid stenosis. N Engl J Med 1991 Aug 15;325(7):445-53.

140 Randomised trial of endarterectomy for recently symptomatic carotid stenosis: final results of the MRC European Carotid Surgery Trial (ECST). Lancet 1998 May 9;351(9113):1379-87.

- Some centers have begun treating carotid disease with angioplasty and stenting rather than with CEA, however the evidence so far suggests that CEA is preferable in most patients[141].

- Since many patients with asymptomatic stenosis are not appropriate surgical candidates, the United States Preventive Services Task Force does not currently recommend screening for carotid stenosis in asymptomatic patients.

SUMMARY AND IMPLICATIONS:

In patients with asymptomatic carotid atherosclerotic disease (stenosis ≥60%), CEA is associated with approximately a 3% perioperative risk. After several years, however, patients who receive surgery have a lower rate of stroke. The decision about whether or not to proceed with surgery depends on patient preference, life expectancy, and the skill of the involved surgeon.

CLINICAL CASE: CAROTID ENDARTERECTOMY FOR ASYMPTOMATIC CAROTID STENOSIS

CASE HISTORY:

An 82 year old man with diabetes, hypertension, and prostate cancer is noted to have a carotid bruit on routine examination. A follow-up ultrasound shows a 70% carotid stenosis.

Based on the results of ACST, how should this patient be treated?

SUGGESTED ANSWER:

The ACST trial showed that CEA can prevent stroke in patients with asymptomatic stenoses ≥60%. However, almost 3% of patients who underwent surgery experienced a perioperative stroke or death, and the risk is likely even higher outside of a research setting. For this reason, surgery is only appropriate among patients who are willing to accept the surgical risk, have a life expectancy of at least several years, and who have access to an experienced and skilled surgeon.

---

141 Davis et al. Carotid-artery stenting in stroke prevention. N Engl J Med. 2010 Jul 1;363(1):80-2.

The elderly man in this vignette has several co-morbidities that suggest he may not be an optimal surgical candidate because his life expectancy may only be a few years. In addition, ACST suggests that patients >75 may not benefit from CEA. For these reasons, this patient is not an optimal candidate for CEA and medical management is likely the best strategy for treating his carotid stenosis.

This case also raises questions about whether patients should be screened for asymptomatic stenosis in the first place. Since many patients with asymptomatic stenosis are not appropriate surgical candidates, the United States Preventive Services Task Force does not currently recommend screening. In routine practice, however, many patients – such as the one in this vignette – do receive screening.

A TRIAL OF ARTHROSCOPIC KNEE SURGERY[142]

"The results ... call into question the widespread use of arthroscopic treatment for osteoarthritis of the knee."

- Kirkely et al.[142]

Research Question: Is arthroscopic surgery for osteoarthritis of the knee effective?

Funding: Canadian Institutes of Health Research

Year Study Began: 1999

Year Study Published: 2008

Study Location: The Kennedy Sport Medicine Clinic, University of Western Ontario, London, Ontario, Canada

Who Was Studied: Adults with osteoarthritis of the knee.

---

142 Kirkley et al. A randomized trial of arthroscopic surgery for osteoarthritis of the knee. N Engl J Med. 2008 Sep 11;359(11):1097-107.

Who Was Excluded: Patients with large meniscal tears, those with inflammatory arthritis, those with prior arthroscopic knee surgery, those with prior major knee trauma, and those with considerable joint deformity.

How Many Patients: 178

Study Overview:

Figure 1: Summary of the Trial's Design

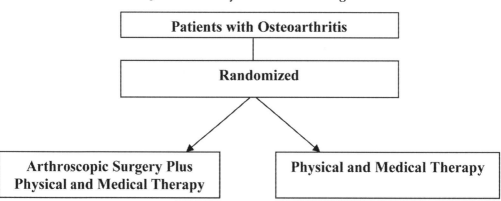

Study Intervention: Patients in the arthroscopy group underwent surgery within 6 weeks of randomization. The surgeon evaluated and irrigated the medial, lateral, and patellofemoral knee compartments, and performed at least one of the following interventions: synovectomy, debridement, or excision of abnormal tissue.

Patients in both the arthroscopy and control groups received physical therapy for one hour a week for 12 weeks, as well as an individualized home exercise program throughout the study period. For pain management, patients were instructed on the use acetaminophen and nonsteroidal anti-inflammatory drugs by an orthopedic surgeon. They were also offered oral glucosamine and intra-articular injections of hyaluronic acid when necessary.

Follow-Up: 2 years

Endpoints: Primary outcome: scores on an osteoarthritis symptom scale (Western Ontario and McMaster Universities Osteoarthritis Index). Secondary outcomes: scores on a scale measuring quality of life (Short Form-36).

RESULTS:

- 3 months after the procedure, patients in the surgery group reported better scores on the arthritis scale, however this benefit was not present at any other point during the study (see Table 1)

- subgroup analyses did not suggest a benefit of surgery for patients with less severe disease, those with more severe radiologic changes, or those with mechanical symptoms of catching or locking

Table 1: The Trial's Key Findings

Outcome	Surgery Group	Control Group	P Value
Mean score on arthritis scale after 2 years[a]	874	897	0.22
Quality of life[b]	37.0	37.2	0.93

[a]Scores range from 0 to 2,400 with higher scores indicating more severe symptoms.
[b]Scores range from 0 to 100 with higher scores indicating a better quality of life.

Criticisms and Limitations: Arthroscopic surgery is still considered to be appropriate in certain situations. For example, most experts believe that patients with symptomatic meniscal tears benefit from arthroscopy. In addition, the subgroup analyses involved only limited numbers of patients, and therefore it is not possible to exclude the possibility of a benefit in certain subgroups such as those with symptoms of catching or locking.

Other Relevant Studies and Information:

- Another widely cited trial randomized patients with osteoarthritis of the knee to arthroscopic debridement, arthroscopic lavage, or a sham procedure[143]. This study also found surgical interventions to be no better than a sham procedure. However this trial has been criticized because only one surgeon participated, it involved mostly older men, and it included patients with considerable joint deformity who might have a poor response to arthroscopic intervention.

---

143 Moseley et al. A controlled trial of arthroscopic surgery for osteoarthritis of the knee. N Engl J Med. 2002 Jul 11;347(2):81-8.

SUMMARY AND IMPLICATIONS:

Despite the fact that patients with osteoarthritis of the knee commonly undergo arthroscopic procedures, surgery does not appear to offer significant benefits. While knee arthroscopy remains appropriate in certain situations (e.g. in patients with symptomatic meniscal tears), most patients with knee pain should be encouraged to treat their symptoms with physical therapy, individualized exercise programs, and pain medications.

CLINICAL CASE: KNEE ARTHROSCOPY

CASE HISTORY:

A 56 year old man presents to the orthopedic clinic with chronic right knee pain. The patient cannot recall any injuries to the knee, but states that it has "been causing problems for years." He has no other joint problems aside from the "usual aches and pains from getting older." On exam, the patient has full range of motion of his right knee and no apparent joint deformities. The knee is mildly to moderately swollen, but there is no warmth or erythema. A recent MRI scan of the knee demonstrated a small meniscal tear and evidence of tendinitis of the knee ligaments, but no ligament tears.

After reading this randomized trial of knee arthroscopy, do you think this patient should undergo knee arthroscopy?

SUGGESTED ANSWER:

The trial of knee arthroscopy showed that patients with osteoarthritis of the knee who were treated with physical therapy, a home exercise program, and acetaminophen and nonsteroidal anti-inflammatory drugs had equivalent outcomes as those who underwent knee arthroscopy. The patient in this vignette is typical of those included in this trial, and thus he should probably be treated with conservative measures rather than arthroscopy. Although some experts believe that patients with symptomatic meniscal tears may benefit from arthroscopy (patients with large meniscal tears were excluded from this trial), this patient's tear is a small one and is unlikely to be contributing to his symptoms. In fact, small meniscal tears are common incidental finding on MRI scans of the knee[144]. However, if conservative measures fail in this patient and his symptoms interfere considerably with his life, he may be a candidate for a knee replacement.

---

144 Englund M, Guermazi A, Gale D, Hunter DJ, Aliabadi P, Clancy M, Felson DT. Incidental meniscal findings on knee MRI in middle-aged and elderly persons. N Engl J Med. 2008 Sep 11;359(11):1108-15.

SURGERY VS. REHABILITATION FOR CHRONIC LOW BACK PAIN:

THE MRC SPINE STABILIZATION TRIAL[145]

"Patients with low back pain ... may obtain similar benefits from an intensive rehabilitation programme as they do from surgery."

- Fairbank et al.[145]

Research Question: Is spinal fusion surgery beneficial in patients with chronic nonspecific low back pain?

Funding: The Medical Research Council of the United Kingdom.

Year Study Began: 1996

Year Study Published: 2005

Study Location: 15 centers in the United Kingdom

Who Was Studied: Adults 18 – 55 with at least 12 months of chronic low back pain (with or without referred pain).

---

145 Fairbank et al. Randomised controlled trial to compare surgical stabilization of the lumbar spine with an intensive rehabilitation programme for patients with chronic lower back pain: the MRC spine stabilisation trial. BMJ. 2005 May 28;330(7502):1233.

Who Was Excluded: Patients who were poor candidates for either of the two treatment strategies, for example patients with spinal infections who required surgery. In addition, patients with previous spinal surgery were excluded.

How Many Patients: 349

Study Overview:

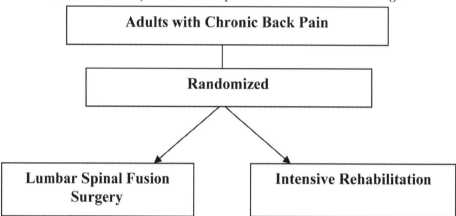

Figure 1: Summary of the MRC Spine Stabilization Trial's Design

Study Intervention: Patients assigned to the surgery group underwent spinal fusion surgery. The surgical technique (e.g. the approach, implant, cages, and bone graft material) "was left to the discretion of the surgeon."

Patients assigned to the intensive rehabilitation group were assigned to a three-week outpatient education and exercise program. The program varied by site, but typically involved 75 hours of therapy along with a follow-up session several weeks afterwards. Physiotherapists led the sessions, and psychologists assisted at most sites as well. In addition, the instructors "used principles of cognitive behavior therapy to identify and overcome fears and unhelpful beliefs that many patients develop when in pain." Patients who did not have an adequate response to rehabilitation were offered surgery.

Follow-Up: 24 months

Endpoints: Primary outcomes: Patient reported pain on the Oswestry low back pain disability index; and patient performance on the shuttle walk test. Secondary outcomes: Scores on the short form 36 (SF-36) general health questionnaire; and surgical complications.

- The Oswestry low back pain disability index is scored from 0 (no disability) to 100 (completely disabled or bedridden)[146]. In the shuttle walk

---

146 Fairbank et al. The Oswestry disability index. Spine. 200;25:2940-53.

test, the distance patients walk during a specified time period and while following instructions is recorded[147].

RESULTS:

- Among patients assigned to the surgery group, 79% received surgery during the study period (21% of patients presumably declined surgery)

- Among patients assigned to the rehabilitation group, 28% received surgery during the study period either because of patient request or because of an inadequate response to rehabilitation

- 12% of patients who underwent surgery experienced a complication such as excessive bleeding, a dural tear, or a vascular injury

- 8% of patients who received surgery required additional surgery after the first operation either to treat a surgical complication or because of persistent symptoms

Table 1: Summary of the Trial's Key Findings

Outcome	Change in Score During Study Period, Surgery Group	Change in Score During Study Period, Rehabilitation Group	P Value[a]
Oswestry Back Pain Score[b]	-12.5	-8.7	0.045
Shuttle Walking Test[c]	+98 meters	+63 meters	0.12
SF-36[d]			
Physical Score	+9.4	+7.6	0.21
Mental Score	+4.2	+3.9	0.90

[a]P value is adjusted for baseline differences between the groups.
[b]A reduction in the back pain score indicates an improvement.
[c]An increase in walking distance on the shuttle walk test indicates an improvement.
[d]An increase in the SF-36 score indicates an improvement.

147 Taylor et al. Reliability and responsiveness of the shuttle walking test in patients with chronic lower back pain. Physiother Res Int. 2001;6:170-8.

- Although scores on the Oswestry back pain scale were significantly better in the surgery group as compared with the rehabilitation group, the difference was very small and is of questionable clinical importance

Criticisms and Limitations: Approximately 20% of patients in the study were lost to follow-up. In addition, there was considerable crossover between the groups (21% of patients in the surgical group never received the surgery while 28% of patients in the rehabilitation group did receive surgery).

The rehabilitation program used in this study was very intensive, and might be too expensive or impractical for many patients. However, whether this intensive rehabilitation program is superior to less intensive programs – or to no rehabilitation at all – is not known.

In the surgery group, the surgical technique was left to the discretion of the surgeon. Surgical outcomes might have been better if the surgical technique had been standardized, though there is considerable controversy about which surgical techniques are best.

Other Relevant Studies and Information:

- Three other trials have compared surgery vs. non-surgical treatment for chronic low back pain, however none was of high methodological quality. A meta-analysis of data from these three trials and the MRC trial concluded: "Surgery may be more efficacious than unstructured non-surgical care for chronic back pain but may not be more efficacious than structured cognitive-behavior therapy. Methodological limitations of the randomized trials prevent firm conclusions."[148]

- Recently, a new surgical technique has been developed for treating patients with chronic low back pain: lumbar disc replacement with an artificial disc. One trial found that disc replacement led to slightly reduced disability after two years of follow-up compared with non-operative care, however the clinical importance of this small difference is uncertain, and it is unclear whether the risks of surgery outweigh the small benefit[149].

- A number of trials have compared surgery (discectomy) vs. non-surgical treatment in patients with severe, persistent sciatica. These trials have

---

148 Mirza and Deyo. Systematic review of randomized trials comparing lumbar fusion surgery to nonoperative care for treatment of chronic back pain. Spine (Phila Pa 1976). 2007;32(7):816.

149 Hellum et al. Surgery with disc prosthesis vs. rehabilitation in patients with low back pain and degenerative disc: two year follow-up of randomised study. BMJ. 2011 May 19;342:d2786.

generally shown equivalent surgical and non-surgical outcomes after a year, but slightly faster improvement in the surgical group[150].

- Guidelines from the American Pain Society recommend that patients with disabling lower back pain lasting more than a year be informed of the risks and benefits of both surgical and non-surgical treatment options. Since both treatments may be equally effective in the long term, the decision about which treatment to pursue should be made by the patient[151].

SUMMARY AND IMPLICATIONS:

The benefit of surgery compared with non-surgical therapy in patients with chronic low back pain remains uncertain. Most patients improve both with and without surgery. Though pain control may be slightly better with surgery, surgical treatment carries risks. Further research on this topic is greatly needed.

CLINICAL CASE: CHRONIC LOW BACK PAIN

CASE HISTORY:

A 48 year old man with low back pain for the past several years is referred to an orthopedic surgeon to consider surgical treatment with lumbar spinal fusion. The symptoms began gradually, and can be quite bothersome, however they do not interfere with his ability to work. The patient denies weakness or bowel or bladder dysfunction. The pain is partially relieved with non-steroidal anti-inflammatory medications.

On physical exam, the patient is obese (body mass index 33). He has a normal neurological exam, and on the straight leg raise test his back pain does not radiate below his knees.

He requests your advice about whether or not to pursue surgery. He feels anxious about "going under the knife" but is willing to do it if you think

---

150 Peul et al. Surgery vs. prolonged conservative treatment for sciatica. N Engl J Med. 2007;356(22):2245.

151 Chou et al. Interventional therapies, surgery, and interdisciplinary rehabilitation for low back pain: an evidence-based clinical practice guideline from the American Pain Society. Spine (Phila Pa 1976). 2009;34(10):1066.

it will help him. Based on the results of the MRC spine stabilization trial, how should you advise him?

SUGGESTED ANSWER:

The benefits of surgical therapy for chronic low back pain remain uncertain. While existing trials suggest that surgery may lead to slightly improved pain control compared with non-surgical therapy, the benefits appear to be small. In addition, surgical treatment carries risks. For these reasons, patients with chronic debilitating low back pain should be informed of the risks and benefits of both surgical and non-surgical treatment options. Using this information, patients should choose the treatment that is most compatible with their personal preferences.

The patient in this vignette has chronic low back pain, however his symptoms do not appear to be debilitating. In addition, his symptoms may improve with weight loss. Moreover, he reports feeling anxious about surgery. For these reasons, he is currently not a good surgical candidate.

If this patient's symptoms worsen, however, surgical treatment could be considered. Prior to receiving surgery, he should be informed of the risks and benefits. In addition, he should be informed that his pain will likely improve considerably over time, even without surgery. The ultimate decision about whether or not to proceed should rest with the patient.

MASTECTOMY VS. LUMPECTOMY FOR INVASIVE BREAST CANCER:

THE B-06 TRIAL[152]

"After 20 years of follow-up, we found no significant difference in overall survival among women who underwent mastectomy and those who underwent lumpectomy with or without post-operative breast irradiation."

- Fisher et al.[152]

Research Question: Do all women with invasive breast cancer require a total mastectomy or is breast conserving therapy (i.e. lumpectomy) appropriate in some women?

---

152 Fisher et al. Twenty-year follow-up of a randomized trial comparing total mastectomy, lumpectomy, and lumpectomy plus irradiation for the treatment of invasive breast cancer. NEJM. 2002 Oct 17;347(16):1233-1241.

Funding: The National Cancer Institute and the Department of Health and Human Services.

Year Study Began: 1976

Year Study Published: 2002

Study Location: 88 centers in the U.S., Canada, and Australia

Who Was Studied: Women with stage I or stage II invasive breast cancer (limited to the ipsilateral breast and axillary nodes) with tumors ≤4 cm.

Who Was Excluded: Women whose tumor had spread beyond the breast and ipsilateral axillary nodes on clinical examination, as well as women with palpable axillary lymph nodes that were not "movable in relation to the chest wall and neurovascular bundle." Additionally, women were excluded if it was not possible to achieve an acceptable cosmetic result with lumpectomy (e.g. if the breast was too small).

How Many Patients: 1851

Study Overview:

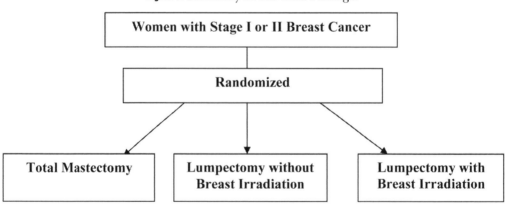

Figure 1: Summary of the Trial's Design

Study Intervention: Patients assigned to the lumpectomy without irradiation group "underwent tumor resection, with removal of sufficient normal breast tissue to ensure both tumor-free [margins] and a satisfactory cosmetic result." In addition, the lower two levels of axillary lymph nodes were removed. If pathology results indicated that the tumor had spread past the margins of the surgical specimen, the patient subsequently underwent total mastectomy.

Patients assigned to the lumpectomy plus breast irradiation group received 50 Gy of irradiation to the breast (but not axilla) following lumpectomy.

Patients assigned to the total mastectomy group received complete resection of the breast and the entire axillary lymph node chain.

All women with positive lymph nodes also received adjuvant systemic chemotherapy with melphalan and fluorouracil.

Follow-Up: 20 years

Endpoints: Disease-free survival, distant disease-free survival, and overall survival.

RESULTS:

- Almost half of the study patients had tumors >2 cm, 38% had positive axillary nodes, and 64% had estrogen receptor positive tumors

- Among patients who underwent lumpectomy, 10% had positive margins on pathology and therefore required a subsequent total mastectomy

- Women who received irradiation following lumpectomy were less likely to have local tumor recurrence in the ipsilateral breast compared with women who received lumpectomy alone (14.3% vs. 39.2%, $P<0.001$)

Table 1: Summary of the Trial's Key Findings

Outcome	Total Mastectomy Group	Lumpectomy without Breast Irradiation Group	Lumpectomy with Breast Irradiation Group	P Value[a]
Disease-Free Survival	36%	35%	35%	0.26
Distant Disease-Free Survival	49%	45%	46%	0.34
Overall Survival	47%	46%	46%	0.57

[a]P value refers to differences among all three groups.

- Lumpectomy followed by irradiation was associated with a slightly lower rate of breast cancer mortality than lumpectomy alone, however this difference was partially offset by an increase in other causes of mortality

Criticisms and Limitations: Approximately 10% of women who received a lumpectomy had positive margins on pathology and subsequently required a mastectomy.

This trial did not exclude the possibility that there are subgroups of women – for example women with large or high grade tumors – in whom total mastectomy leads to better outcomes than lumpectomy.

Other Relevant Studies and Information:

- Other trials have also demonstrated the equivalency of breast conserving therapy and total mastectomy[153,154].

- Other studies also confirm the finding that breast irradiation following lumpectomy reduces the risk of local cancer recurrence in the ipsilateral breast and lowers breast-cancer related mortality[155]. For this reason, most women receiving breast conserving therapy also receive breast irradiation. However, breast irradiation appears to be associated with a slight increase in non-breast cancer related mortality that partially offsets the reduction in breast cancer related mortality[155].

- Currently, breast conserving therapy is considered to be the preferred treatment for early stage breast cancer[156]. Still, many women with early stage breast cancer who are appropriate candidates for lumpectomy are only offered the option of total mastectomy[157].

SUMMARY AND IMPLICATIONS:

In women with early stage breast cancer, total mastectomy does not reduce either disease-free survival or overall survival compared with breast conserving therapy (i.e. lumpectomy). Breast irradiation following lumpectomy reduces the risk of local cancer recurrence and leads to a small

153 Veronesi et al. Twenty-year follow-up of a randomized study comparing breast-conserving surgery with radical mastectomy for early breast cancer. NEJM. 2002 Oct 17;347(16):1227-1232.

154 Early Breast Cancer Trialists' Collaborative Group. Effects of radiotherapy and surgery in early breast cancer: an overview of the randomized trials. NEJM 1995;333:1444-55.

155 Clarke et al. Effects of radiotherapy and of differences in the extent of surgery for early breast cancer on local recurrence and 15-year survival: an overview of the randomised trials. Lancet. 2005;366(9503):2087.

156 NIH Consensus Development Conference statement on the treatment of early-stage breast cancer. Oncology (Williston Park) 1991; 5:120.

157 Morrow M et al. Factors predicting the use of breast-conserving therapy in stage I and II breast carcinoma. J Clin Oncol 2001;19:2254-62.

reduction in breast cancer related mortality, but this reduction is partially offset by an increase in death from other causes.

CLINICAL CASE: TOTAL MASTECTOMY VS. LUMPECTOMY

CASE HISTORY:

A 58 year old woman is referred to a breast surgeon with newly diagnosed breast cancer. The tumor was detected after the patient noticed a new lump in her right breast.

On examination, the woman is noted to have a 5 cm mass in the upper, outer quadrant of her right breast. She also is noted to have palpable right axillary lymph nodes that are mobile in relation to her chest wall. She has no evidence of lymph node involvement elsewhere, nor does she have evidence of distant metastatic disease. (These findings are consistent with stage II breast cancer since the tumor is confined to the right breast and to mobile right axillary lymph nodes.)

As the patient's surgeon, you must explain the options for treating this patient. Based on the results of the B-06 trial, what should you tell her?

SUGGESTED ANSWER:

Since this patient has early stage breast cancer (stage II), she is an appropriate candidate for surgical removal of the tumor (patients with stage IV breast cancer, and many patients with stage III breast cancer, are treated with systemic therapy rather than surgery). In addition, based on the results of the B-06 trial and other studies, breast conserving surgery is the preferred surgical option for most women with early stage breast cancer.

This patient has a large tumor (5 cm), however, and in the B-06 trial, only women with tumors ≤4 cm were offered the option of breast conserving surgery. Similarly, none of the other trials comparing total mastectomy with breast conserving surgery included women with tumors >4 – 5 cm. Even so, the presence of a tumor ≥5 cm is not considered to be a contraindication to breast conserving surgery as long as the surgeon feels it is possible to remove the tumor with clean surgical margins and to achieve a good cosmetic result. Therefore, this patient should still be considered for breast conserving surgery as long as the surgeon feels that successful treatment with lumpectomy is possible.

Finally, as in all situations, the decision about whether this woman should receive a total mastectomy vs. breast conserving surgery should take into account the patient's personal preferences. Despite the data showing the equivalency of breast conserving surgery and mastectomy, some women opt for total mastectomies for psychological reasons.

LONG TERM IMPACT OF BARIATRIC SURGERY:

THE SWEDISH OBESE SUBJECTS STUDY[158,159]

"In this prospective, controlled study, we showed that bariatric surgery in obese subjects was associated with a reduction in overall mortality ...."

- *Sjöström* et al.[158]

Research Question: Does bariatric surgery in obese individuals reduce mortality?

Funding: Hoffmann-La Roche, AstraZeneca, Cederroth, and the Swedish Research Council.

Year Study Began: 1987

Year Study Published: 2007

158 Sjöström et al. Effects of bariatric surgery on mortality in Swedish obese subjects. N Engl J Med. 2007 Aug 23;357(8):741-52.

159 Bray G. The missing link – lose weight, live longer. N Engl J Med. 2007 Aug 23;357(8):818-20.

Study Location: 25 surgical departments and 480 primary health care centers in Sweden

Who Was Studied: Adults 37-60 years old with a body mass index (BMI) of 34 or higher in men and 38 or higher in women.

Who Was Excluded: Patients who were not eligible for surgery, and those with a myocardial infarction or stroke within the previous 6 months.

How Many Patients: 4,047

Study Overview:

Figure 1: Summary of the Study's Design

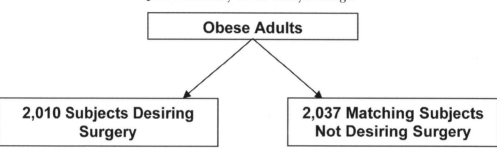

- The subjects were not randomized into surgical and non-surgical groups. Rather, obese individuals desiring bariatric surgery were recruited, and for each enrolled surgical subject, a matched control patient who was eligible for surgery but not desiring it was recruited. Patients in both groups were followed prospectively, making this a prospective controlled study.

Study Intervention: Approximately 19% of the patients who desired surgery underwent gastric banding, 68% underwent vertical banded gastroplasty, and 13% underwent gastric bypass.

The matching control patients – who were identified using 18 matching variables – received standard nonsurgical treatment for obesity. This varied from "sophisticated lifestyle intervention and behavior modification to no treatment whatsoever."

Follow-Up: Mean of 10.9 years

Endpoints: Mortality rates were compared between subjects who underwent surgery and those who didn't. Both unadjusted mortality rates, as well as mortality rates adjusted for differences between the groups (e.g. differences in age, smoking status, rates of diabetes, and weight) were examined.

RESULTS:

- the average BMI of patients opting for surgery was 41.8 vs. 40.9 among patients not desiring surgery (P<0.001)

- patients in the surgery group were younger (46.1 years vs. 47.4 years, P<0.001) and more likely to be smokers (27.9% vs. 20.2%, P<0.001) than patients in the control group

- within 90 days of surgery, 0.25% of patients in the surgery group died vs. 0.10% in the control group during the same time period

Table 1: Percentage Change in Body Weight After 10 Years

Controls	Gastric Bypass	Vertical Banded Gastroplasty	Gastric Banding
+2%	-25%	-16%	-14%

Table 2: Mortality Rates

Surgery Group	Controls	Hazard Ratio	P Value
5.0%	6.3%	0.76	0.04

- after adjustment for baseline differences between groups, mortality rates remained significantly lower among patients who opted for surgery (P=0.01)

Criticisms and Limitations: The major shortcoming of this study is that it was not a randomized trial, and therefore the lower mortality among surgical patients may have resulted from factors other than the procedure itself. For example, it is possible that patients who opted for surgery were of higher socioeconomic status than those who didn't. As a result, they may have lived longer as a result of having better access to healthcare services. The authors attempted to control for differences between groups but it is never possible to adjust for all differences.

In addition, newer techniques for bariatric surgery – including laparoscopy – have become available since this study was conducted, and therefore surgical complication rates may now be lower than reported in this study. Furthermore, the study was too small to determine which patients (e.g. older vs. younger) benefit most from surgery, or whether less invasive procedures like gastric banding or vertical banded gastroplasty are as effective as gastric bypass.

Finally, the absolute benefit of bariatric surgery for reducing mortality was quite modest: 5.0% mortality among surgery patients vs. 6.3% among controls.

Other Relevant Studies and Information:

• A previous analysis of the Swedish Obese Subjects Study showed favorable effects of bariatric surgery on the rates and progression of diabetes, hypertriglyceridemia, hypertension, hyperuricemia, and on health-related quality of life[160]. More recently, results from the study suggest that bariatic surgery is associated with a reduction in the incidence of cancer among women[161], as well as cardiovascular events and cardiovascular death[162].

• A retrospective cohort study published in the same issue of the *New England Journal of Medicine* also showed a reduction in mortality rates among obese patients who underwent gastric bypass surgery vs. those who were treated non-surgically[163].

SUMMARY AND IMPLICATIONS:

Though it was not a randomized trial, the Swedish Obese Subjects Study is the best demonstration yet that bariatric surgery (gastric banding, vertical banded gastroplasty, and gastric bypass) leads to long-term weight loss and a modest but detectable reduction in all-cause mortality in patients with severe obesity. The study also showed favorable effects of bariatric surgery on cardiovascular disease, diabetes, hypertriglyceridemia, hypertension, hyperuricemia, health-related quality of life, and on the incidence of cancer among women.

---

160 Sjostrom et al. Lifestyle, diabetes, and cardiovascular risk factors 10 years after bariatric surgery. N Engl J Med 2004;351:2683-2693.

161 Sjostrom et al. Effects of bariatric surgery on cancer incidence in obese patients in Sweden (Swedish Obese Subjects Study): a prospective, controlled intervention trial. Lancet Oncol. 2009 Jul;10(7):653-62.

162 Sjöström et al. Bariatric surgery and long-term cardiovascular events. JAMA. 2012 Jan 4;307(1):56-65.

163 Adams et al. Long-term mortality after gastric bypass surgery. N Engl J Med 2007;357:753-761.

CLINICAL CASE: BARIATRIC SURGERY

CASE HISTORY:

A 54 year old man with a BMI of 36 visits your clinic to discuss management of his diabetes. He is on high doses of insulin and metformin, but his HbA1c remains elevated at 8.4%. He has tried numerous times to lose weight by dieting, but hasn't had any long term success. He is very committed to improving his health, but feels increasingly frustrated with dieting.

You decide to discuss the possibility of bariatric surgery with this patient. Based on the results of the Swedish Obese Subjects study, what can you tell him about the potential benefits?

SUGGESTED ANSWER:

You could explain to the patient that bariatric surgery – including gastric banding, vertical banded gastroplasty, and gastric bypass – has been shown to produce long-term weight loss and a modest but detectable reduction in all-cause mortality in patients with severe obesity. Bariatric surgery also leads to favorable effects on obesity-related medical problems including cardiovascular disease, diabetes, elevated lipid levels, hypertension, and perhaps cancer. In addition, patients who undergo surgery are likely to experience an improvement in quality of life.

Surgery carries with it risks, however. In the Swedish Obese Subjects Study, 0.25% of patients (1 in 400) died within 90 days of surgery. In comparison, only 0.10% of control patients (1 in 1,000) died during the same time period.

While the decision to undergo bariatric surgery is of course a personal one and involves multiple different factors, you should recommend that your patient learn about bariatric surgery. Ideally, you should refer him to a bariatric surgery center to meet with bariatric surgery specialists.

SECTION 4:

OBSTETRICS

THE CANADIAN MULTICENTER POST-TERM PREGNANCY TRIAL (CMPPT)[164]

"[I]nducing labor in women with post-term pregnancies results in a decrease in the rate of cesarean section as compared with serial antenatal monitoring ...."

- Hannah et al.[164]

Research Question: Should labor be induced in women with post-term pregnancies?

Funding: The Medical Research Council of Canada.

Year Study Began: 1985

Year Study Published: 1992

Study Location: 22 hospitals in Canada

164 Hannah et al. Induction of labor as compared with serial antenatal monitoring in post-term pregnancy. NEJM. 1992 Jun 11;326(24):1587-1592.

Who Was Studied: Pregnant women whose pregnancies had reached at least 41 weeks' gestation. Women were also required to have a live singleton fetus.

Who Was Excluded: Women were excluded if the cervix was dilated ≥3 cm, if the gestational age was ≥44 weeks, if the fetus was non-cephalic (i.e. breech or shoulder presentation), if the woman had serious medical problems such as diabetes or preeclampsia, if the fetus showed signs of a lethal congenital anomaly, if an urgent delivery was necessary (e.g. fetal distress), or if a vaginal delivery was contraindicated (e.g. placenta previa).

How Many Patients: 3407

Study Overview:

Figure 1: Summary of the CMPPT's Design

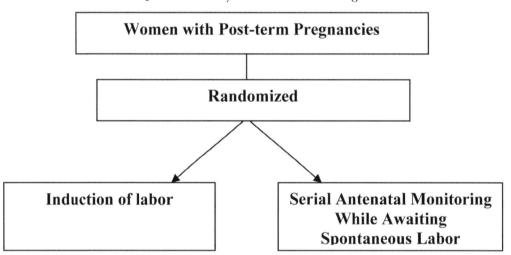

Study Intervention: Women assigned to the induction group were induced within four days of enrollment. Prostaglandin E_2 gel was used to "ripen" the cervix if necessary, and this treatment could be repeated up to two additional times. In women who did not receive the gel, or if the prostaglandin administration did not induce labor, an oxytocin infusion, amniotomy, or both were used to induce labor.

Women assigned to the monitoring group were instructed to count fetal kicks over a two-hour period each day and to contact their physician for non-stress testing if they felt fewer than six kicks during this time period. (A non-stress test is a 20-30 minute test in which the fetal heart rate and heart rate reactivity are monitored along with fetal movements and uterine contractions.) In addition, these women received regular non-stress tests three times per week and ultrasounds two to three times per week to assess the amniotic-fluid volume. The fetus was delivered immediately, either by inducing labor or by cesarean section, if the non-stress test was concerning, if the amniotic fluid volume was low (a pocket <3 cm), if other complications developed, or if the gestational age reached 44 weeks.

In both groups, the attending physician determined whether the fetus would be delivered vaginally or by cesarean section based on the clinical circumstances.

Follow-Up: From maternal enrollment until hospital discharge of the baby

Endpoints: Primary outcomes: Perinatal mortality (stillbirths and neonatal deaths before discharge, excluding deaths due to lethal congenital anomalies); and neonatal morbidity (e.g. an Apgar score <7 at 5 minutes, coma or lethargy, or the need for mechanical ventilation). Secondary outcome: Cesarean section rate.

RESULTS:

- Within a week of enrollment, 94.9% of women in the induction group had delivered their babies vs. 74.0% in the monitoring group (P<0.001)

- Women in both groups were more likely to receive a cesarean section if they were nulliparous, older, had a less fully dilated cervix, were black, or were in the racial category "other"

Table 1: Summary of CMPPT's Key Findings

Outcome	Induction Group	Monitoring Group	P Value
Perinatal Mortality	0.0%[a]	0.1%[a]	Not significant[b]
Neonatal Morbidity			
Apgar score <7 at 5 minutes	1.1%	1.2%	Not significant[b]
Coma or lethargy	1.0%	0.9%	Not significant[b]
Need for mechanical ventilation	0.5%	0.6%	Not significant[b]
Cesarean Section Rate	21.2%	24.5%	0.03
Cesarean Section Rate Due to Fetal Distress	5.7%	8.3%	0.003

[a]After excluding two infants with lethal congenital anomalies from the analysis, there were no perinatal deaths in the induction group. There were two stillbirths and no neonatal deaths in the monitoring group.
[b]Actual P value not reported.

- There were no significant differences in postpartum maternal morbidity between the groups

Criticisms and Limitations: The trial was underpowered to detect small differences between labor induction vs. serial monitoring on perinatal outcomes.

Other Relevant Studies and Information:

- Other studies are generally consistent with CMPTT[165], however some have suggested slightly higher rates of perinatal mortality[166] and neonatal morbidity with serial monitoring as compared with induction[165].

---

165 Caughey et al. Systematic review: elective induction of labor vs. expectant management of pregnancy. Ann Intern Med. 2009;151(4):252.

166 Gülmezoglu et al. Induction of labour for improving birth outcomes for women at or beyond term. Cochrane Database Syst Rev. 2006 Oct 18;(4):CD004945.

- A cost analysis involving data from the CMPTT trial suggested that labor induction is less costly than serial monitoring[167].

- Studies have suggested worse perinatal outcomes with labor induction before 39 weeks' gestation[168].

SUMMARY AND IMPLICATIONS:

In women with post-term (≥41 weeks) pregnancies, induction of labor results in a slight decrease in the rate of cesarean section compared with serial monitoring, and appears to be a less costly strategy. CMPTT did not show a significant effect of induction vs. serial monitoring on perinatal mortality or neonatal morbidity, however a pooled analysis of data from CMPTT and other studies suggests that induction leads to a small but significant benefit with respect to these outcomes. Because of these findings, obstetricians often encourage labor induction after 41 weeks. Since the differences in outcomes between induction vs. serial monitoring are small, however, either strategy is appropriate.

CLINICAL CASE: MANAGEMENT OF POST-TERM PREGNANCIES

CASE HISTORY:

A 30 year old G1P0 woman without any medical problems reaches the 41st week of her pregnancy. She feels well, and reports frequent fetal movements. In addition, a non-stress test is reassuring, and her amniotic fluid level is normal.

The patient's obstetrician asks her if she would like to be induced. She appears hesitant.

Based on the results of CMPPT, should the obstetrician try to persuade her to undergo induction?

---

167 Goeree et al. Cost-effectiveness of induction of labour vs. serial antenatal monitoring in the Canadian Multicentre Postterm Pregnancy Trial. CMAJ. 1995. May 1;152(9):1445-50.

168 Clark et al. Neonatal and maternal outcomes associated with elective term delivery. Am J Obstet Gynecol. 2009;200(2):156.e1.

SUGGESTED ANSWER:

The CMPPT trial showed a small but significant reduction in the rate of cesarean section with induction compared with serial monitoring. Studies have also suggested a small but significant reduction in the risk of perinatal mortality and neonatal morbidity with induction. Since the absolute risks of these complications are very small, however, serial monitoring is an appropriate strategy for managing post-term pregnancies in women who prefer this approach.

The obstetrician in this vignette probably should not try too hard to persuade his patient to be induced. If the patient opts for serial monitoring, she should be monitored regularly (twice a week) with non-stress testing, amniotic fluid measurements by ultrasound, and/or other tests such as the biophysical profile[169]. If she does not go into labor spontaneously by 42-43 weeks' gestation, most obstetricians would recommend induction more vigorously.

---

169 American College of Obstetricians and Gynecologists. Antepartum fetal surveillance. ACOG practice bulletin #9. Amercan College of Obstetricians and Gynecologists, Washington, DC 1999.

ANTEPARTUM GLUCOCORTICOIDS IN PREMATURE LABOR[170]

"Relatively brief intrauterine exposure of human infants to pharmacological doses of betamethasone was associated with a substantial reduction in the incidence of [respiratory distress syndrome] which was particularly marked in the most immature group."

- Liggins and Howie[170]

Research Question: Can respiratory distress syndrome (RDS) be prevented in neonates by administering glucocorticoids to women at risk for premature labor?

Funding: The Medical Research Council of New Zealand.

Year Study Began: 1969

---

170 Liggins GD and Howie RN. A controlled trial of antepartum glucocorticoid treatment for prevention of respiratory distress syndrome in premature infants. Pediatrics. 1972;50:515-525.

Year Study Published: 1972

Study Location: National Women's Hospital, Auckland, New Zealand

Who Was Studied: Women "admitted in premature labor at 24 – 36 weeks [gestation] or in whom premature delivery before 37 weeks was planned because of an obstetrical complication."

Who Was Excluded: Women in whom the treating obstetrician felt that glucocorticoid treatment was contraindicated as well as women who gave birth shortly after admission to the hospital.

How Many Patients: 282 mothers

Study Overview:

Figure 1: Summary of the Trial's Design

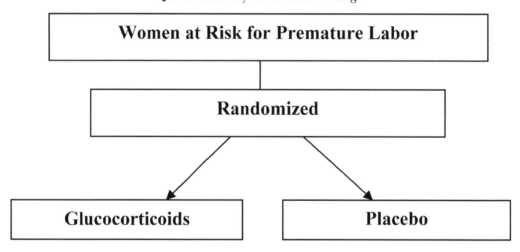

Study Intervention: Women assigned to the glucocorticoid group received an intramuscular injection of betamethasone 12 mg followed by a second dose 24 hours later unless delivery had already occurred.

Women assigned to the placebo group received placebo injections according to the same schedule.

When women in either group presented in spontaneous labor, the treating obstetrician attempted to delay delivery by 48 – 72 hours with tocolytics (either intravenous ethanol or salbutamol) in order to provide time for the betamethasone (or placebo) to have its effect. If spontaneous rupture of the fetal membranes was present, "attempted suppression of labor was limited to 48 hours" and women were treated with antibiotics.

Women in both groups who were scheduled for premature deliveries because of obstetrical complications received the first dose of betamethasone or placebo three days prior to the planned induction.

Follow-Up: Neonatal outcomes were monitored for the first 7 days of life

Endpoints: Respiratory distress syndrome; Apgar scores; and perinatal mortality.

- In order to qualify as having RDS, an infant was required to have both clinical signs (grunting and chest retraction) and radiological signs ("fine generalized granularity of lung fields with air bronchogram") of the syndrome.

RESULTS:

- The reasons for premature labor included: spontaneous premature labor (76%), and planned premature labor for fetal malformations (5%), Rh hemolytic disease of the newborn (7%), pre-eclampsia (11%), and placenta previa (1%)

- Betamethasone therapy was not associated with any maternal complications, nor was it associated with fetal or neonatal complications (infections, hypoglycemia, jaundice, or diarrhea)

Table 1: Summary of the Trial's Key Findings[a]

Outcome	Betamethasone Group	Placebo Group	P Value
Incidence of RDS[b]	9.0%	25.8%	0.003
Apgar Scores at 5 Minutes	8.0	7.5	Not significant[c]
Total Perinatal Mortality	6.4%	18.0%	0.02
Fetal Deaths	3.2%	3.0%	Not significant[c]
Early Neonatal Deaths	3.2%	15.0%	0.01

[a]Data are only for the subgroup of infants born to mothers with spontaneous premature labor (76% of all mothers in the study).
[b]Among all live births.
[c]Actual p value not listed.

- betamethasone was more effective in preventing RDS and perinatal mortality among mothers who gave birth at least 24 hours after trial entry than among mothers who gave birth within the first 24 hours

- betamethasone was more effective in preventing RDS and perinatal mortality among infants who were delivered prior to 32 weeks of gestation than among infants who were delivered after 32 weeks (presumably because perinatal complications are much less common after 32 weeks of gestation)

Criticisms and Limitations: The trial only included a small number of women who underwent planned labor induction due to obstetrical complications and therefore it is not possible to draw firm conclusions about glucocorticoids in this subgroup. Subsequent studies have shown glucocorticoids to be beneficial in these women, however.

Other Relevant Studies and Information:

- Numerous other studies have confirmed the benefits of glucocorticoids in preventing neonatal RDS and perinatal mortality when given to women at risk for pre-mature labor[171]

- Subsequent studies have also demonstrated that glucocorticoids reduce the risk of neonatal intraventricular hemorrhage, necrotizing enterocolitis, and systemic infections when given to women at risk for pre-mature labor[172]

- Guidelines from professional organizations and from the National Institutes of Health[173] recommend administration of glucocorticoids to all mothers at risk for premature delivery prior to 34 weeks of gestation; two doses of intramuscular betamethasone 12 mg are typically given 24 hours apart

---

171 Crowley P. Prophylactic glucocorticoids for preterm birth. Cochrane Database Syst Rev. 2000;(2):CD000065. Review.

172 Roberts D and Dalziel S Antenatal glucocorticoids for accelerating fetal lung maturation for women at risk of preterm birth. Cochrane Database Syst Rev. 2006;3:CD004454.

173 Report on the Consensus Development Conference on the Effect of Glucocorticoids for Fetal Maturation on Perinatal Outcomes. U.S. Department of Health and Human Services, Public Health Service, NIH Pub No. 95-3784, November 1994.

SUMMARY AND IMPLICATIONS:

Administration of antenatal betamethasone to women at risk for pre-mature labor is effective in preventing respiratory distress syndrome and perinatal mortality in neonates. The treatment is most effective among women experiencing premature labor prior to 32 weeks of gestation and when the betamethasone is given at least 24 hours before delivery.

CLINICAL CASE: ANTEPARTUM GLUCOCORTICOIDS IN PREMATURE LABOR

CASE HISTORY:

A G1P0 woman is admitted to the hospital in premature labor at 34 weeks gestation. Thus far, she has had an uncomplicated pregnancy. She is well-appearing, and the fetal heart tracing is reassuring.

Based on the results of this trial, should you administer betamethasone to this patient to promote fetal lung maturation?

SUGGESTED ANSWER:

This trial showed that betamethasone is most effective in preventing perinatal complications prior to 32 weeks of gestation. Most guidelines recommend that glucocorticoids be given to all mothers at risk for premature delivery prior to 34 weeks gestation, however.

Thus, this woman who is in premature labor at 34 weeks gestation is on the cusp of needing glucocorticoids. Treatment could be considered but is not clearly indicated.

SECTION 5:

PEDIATRICS

TREATMENT OF ACUTE OTITIS MEDIA IN CHILDREN[174]

"[A]mong children 6 to 23 months of age with acute otitis media, treatment with amoxicillin-clavulanate for 10 days affords a measurable short-term benefit ... The benefit must be weighed against concern not only about the side effects of the medication but also about the ... emergence of bacterial resistance. These considerations underscore the need to restrict treatment to children whose illness is diagnosed with the use of stringent criteria."

- Hoberman et al.[174]

Research Question: Should children under two years of age with acute otitis media be treated immediately with antibiotics?

Funding: The National Institute of Allergy and Infectious Diseases

Year Study Began: 2006

---

174 Hoberman et al. Treatment of acute otitis media in children under 2 years of age. NEJM. 2011; 364(2):105-115.

Year Study Published: 2011

Study Location: The Children's Hospital of Pittsburgh and Armstrong Pediatrics (a private practice in Pennsylvania)

Who Was Studied: Children 6 - 23 months of age with acute otitis media. To qualify, children were required to have:

- Onset of acute otitis media symptoms within the previous 48 hours

- A score of ≥3 on the Acute Otitis Media Severity of Symptoms scale (AOM-SOS), which is scored from 0 – 14 based on parental reports of: "tugging of ears, crying, irritability, difficulty sleeping, diminished activity, diminished appetite, and fever"

- Middle-ear effusion

- Moderate or severe "bulging of the tympanic membrane or slight bulging accompanied by either otalgia or marked erythema of the membrane"

Who Was Excluded: Children with another illness such as pneumonia or cystic fibrosis, those who had not yet received at least two doses of the pneumococcal conjugate vaccine, those with an allergy to amoxicillin, those with recent antibiotic exposure, and those with a ruptured tympanic membrane.

How Many Patients: 291

Study Overview:

Figure 1: Summary of the Trial's Design

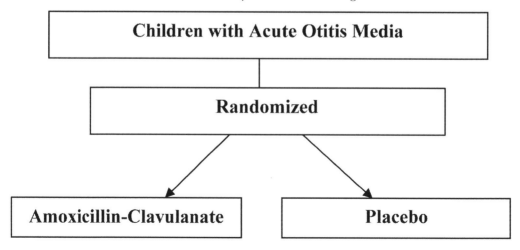

Study Intervention: Children assigned to the antibiotic group received amoxicillin-clavulanate in two divided doses for 10 days (total daily dose 90 mg/kg of amoxicillin and 6.4 mg/kg of clavulanate). Children assigned to the control group received a placebo suspension twice daily for 10 days.

Follow-Up: Evaluations were conducted at various time intervals during the first 21-25 days after enrollment.

Endpoints: Primary outcomes: Time to symptom resolution; and symptom burden. Secondary outcomes: clinical failure; adverse events; and health care resource utilization.

RESULTS:

- at baseline, the mean AOM-SOS score was 7.8, and 52% of children had bilateral disease; in addition, 72% of children had moderate or severe bulging of the tympanic membrane

Table 1: Summary of the Trial's Key Findings

Outcome	Antibiotics Group	Control Group	P Value
Initial Symptom Resolution[a]			
Day 2	35%	28%	0.14[c]
Day 4	61%	54%	
Day 7	80%	74%	
Sustained Symptom Resolution[b]			
Day 2	20%	14%	0.04[c]
Day 4	41%	36%	
Day 7	67%	53%	
Symptom Burden[d]	2.79	3.42	0.01
Clinical Failure[e]			
At or before day 4-5	4%	23%	<0.001
At or before day 10-12	16%	51%	<0.001
Infection-related Complications			
Mastoiditis	0%	1%	Non-significant[f]
Tympanic membrane perforation	1%	5%	Non-significant[f]

Outcome	Antibiotics Group	Control Group	P Value
Antibiotic-related Complications			
Diarrhea	25%	15%	0.05
Diaper rash	51%	35%	0.008
Oral thrush	5%	1%	Non-significant[f]

[a]Defined as AOM-SOS score of 0 or 1.
[b]Defined as two consecutive recordings of an AOM-SOS score of 0 or 1.
[c]For overall trend.
[d]Defined as the mean weighted AOM-SOS scores over first 7 days of follow-up.
[e]Defined at days 4-5 as a "lack of substantial improvement in symptoms, a worsening of signs on otoscopic examination, or both" and at days 10-12 as "the failure to achieve complete or nearly complete resolution of symptoms and otoscopic signs" with the exception of middle ear effusion.
[f]Actual p value not reported.

- treatment with amoxicillin-clavulanate resulted in the greatest absolute benefit among children with the most severe infections (AOM-SOS score >8)

- there were no differences between the antibiotic vs. control groups with regard to the use of acetaminophen or the utilization of health care resources

Criticisms and Limitations: The children in this study had acute otitis media diagnosed using stringent criteria. The findings are not applicable to children with an "uncertain" diagnosis of otitis media (e.g. those with no clear bulging of the tympanic membrane).

The authors defined clinical failure based (in part) on findings on otoscopic exam, however it is uncertain whether children who become asymptomatic but have otoscopic findings of persistent middle-ear infection are at increased risk for recurrent symptomatic illness.

The authors chose amoxicillin-clavulanate for this study as it has been shown to be the most effective oral antibiotic for acute otitis media. Guidelines from the American Academy of Pediatrics and the American Academy of Family Practice recommend amoxicillin as first-line therapy, however.

Other Relevant Studies and Information:

- Other trials comparing immediate antibiotics vs. watchful waiting in children with acute otitis media have also generally suggested that antibiotics lead to modestly faster resolution of symptoms but increased rates of side effects (particularly diarrhea and rash)[175,176,177]

- Data on the impact of antibiotic therapy on antimicrobial resistance are limited, however one study suggests that antibiotics lead to an increase in the rates of nasopharyngeal carriage of resistant *Streptococcus pneumoniae*[178]

- Guidelines from the American Academy of Pediatrics and the American Academy of Family Practice recommend antibiotics in the following circumstances[179]:

  ➤ all children <6 months with suspected otitis media
  ➤ children 6 months – 2 years when the symptoms are severe
  ➤ children >2 years if the diagnosis is certain and the illness is severe

The guidelines state that watchful waiting with close observation may be considered for:

  ➤ children 6 months – 2 years in whom the symptoms are not severe and the diagnosis is uncertain
  ➤ children >2 years in whom either the diagnosis is uncertain or the symptoms are not severe

SUMMARY AND IMPLICATIONS:

Among children <2 with stringently diagnosed acute otitis media, amoxicillin-clavulanate hastened the resolution of symptoms, reduced the overall symptom burden, and resulted in a lower rate of treatment failure but was associated with side effects (diarrhea and diaper dermatitis). Guidelines from the American Academy of Pediatrics (listed above) provide recommendations regarding which children with suspected acute otitis media should receive antibiotics vs. watchful waiting with close observation.

175 Glasziou et al. Antibiotics for acute otitis media in children. Cochrane Database Syst Rev. 2004.

176 Coker et al. Diagnosis, microbial epidemiology, and antibiotic treatment of acute otitis media in children: a systematic review. JAMA. 2010;304(19):2161.

177 Tähtinen et al. A placebo-controlled trial of antimicrobial treatment for acute otitis media. N Engl J Med. 2011 Jan 13;364(2):116-26.

178 McCormick et al. Nonsevere acute otitis media: a clinical trial comparing outcomes of watchful waiting vs. immediate antibiotic treatment. Pediatrics. 2005;115(6):1455.

179 American Academy of Pediatrics Subcommittee on Management of Acute Otitis Media. Diagnosis and management of acute otitis media. Pediatrics. 2004;113(5):1451.

CLINICAL CASE: ANTIBIOTICS FOR ACUTE OTITIS MEDIA

CASE HISTORY:

An 18 month old girl is brought to the office by her father with 36 hours of rhinorrhea, irritability, and a low grade fever (99.5 °F). She has been eating normally, but awoke several times the previous night crying.

On exam, the girl is well-appearing with evidence of rhinorrhea and a temperature of 99.2 °F. Otherwise her vital signs are within normal limits. You attempt to look in her ears but have difficulty making her stay still. From the brief look you get, it appears she may have a middle ear effusion in her right ear and perhaps a slightly erythematous tympanic membrane without bulging.

Based on the results of this trial, should you prescribe this girl an antibiotic for the treatment of acute otitis media?

SUGGESTED ANSWER:

The above-described trial demonstrated that antibiotics are effective in children under 2 years of age with acute otitis media diagnosed using stringent criteria.

The girl in this vignette has an uncertain diagnosis of acute otitis media (her symptoms could be due entirely to a viral upper respiratory infection). In addition, her symptoms are relatively mild. Thus, the results of the trial do not necessarily apply to this patient.

Guidelines from the American Academy of Pediatrics and the American Academy of Family Practice indicate that watchful waiting with close observation – rather than immediate antibiotics – can be considered for children 6 months – 2 years with an uncertain diagnosis of otitis media and mild symptoms. Thus, the girl in this vignette would be a good candidate for watchful waiting. If the watchful waiting strategy is chosen, the father should be instructed to call the office immediately should his daughter's condition worsen or not improve within a few days (if her condition worsens, she would likely need to be treated with antibiotics). Someone from the clinic might also call the family a couple of days later to make sure the girl is improving.

A TRIAL OF EARLY EAR TUBE PLACEMENT IN CHILDREN WITH PERSISTENT OTITIS MEDIA[180]

"In children younger than three years of age who have persistent otitis media, prompt insertion of tympanostomy tubes does not measurably improve developmental outcomes ..."

- Paradise et al.[180]

Research Question: Does early placement of ear tubes in young children with persistent otitis media lead to improved developmental outcomes (i.e. speech and language skills, cognition, and psychosocial development)?

---

180 Paradise et al. Effect of early or delayed insertion of tympanostomy tubes for persistent otitis media on developmental outcomes at the age of three years. N Engl J Med. 2001 Apr 19;344(16):1179-1187.

Funding: The National Institute for Child Health and Human Development, the Agency for Healthcare Research and Quality, and two pharmaceutical companies.

Year Study Began: 1991

Year Study Published: 2001

Study Location: 8 sites in the Pittsburgh area (2 hospital clinics and 6 private group practices)

Who Was Studied: Children between the ages of 2 months and 3 years who had a "substantial" middle ear effusion persisting for at least 90 days in the case of bilateral effusion or 135 days in the case of unilateral effusion despite antibiotic therapy. In addition, children with intermittent effusion meeting certain criteria (e.g. bilateral effusion lasting 67% of a 180-day period) were eligible. Children were identified for the trial from a group of volunteer infants who underwent regular (at least monthly) ear exams.

Who Was Excluded: Children with a low birth weight (<5 lb), those with a major congenital abnormality, and those with other serious illnesses.

How Many Patients: 429

Study Overview:

Figure 1: Summary of the Trial's Design

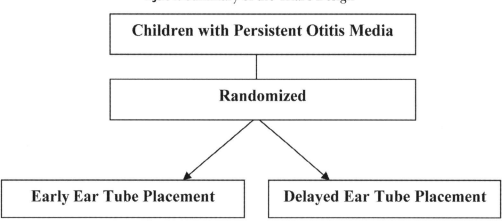

Study Intervention: Children assigned to early ear tube placement were scheduled for the procedure "as soon as practicable."

Those assigned to delayed placement received the procedure only if a bilateral effusion persisted for an additional 6 months or if a unilateral effusion persisted for an additional 9 months. Children in the delayed placement group also received ear tubes at any point if their parents requested it.

Follow-Up: 3 years

Endpoints: The authors evaluated the following developmental outcomes:

- Cognition, as assessed using the McCarthy Scales of Children's Abilities[181]

- Receptive language, as assessed using the Peabody Picture Vocabulary Test[182]

- Expressive language, as assessed by analyzing 15-minute samples of each child's spontaneous conversation (the authors recorded the number of different words, the mean length of utterances, and the percentage of consonants correct for each child)

- Parental stress, as assessed using parental responses to the Parenting Stress Index, Short Form[183]

- Child behavior, as assessed using parental responses to the Child Behavior Checklist[184]

In addition, the authors estimated the number of days that ear effusion persisted in the early placement vs. delayed placement groups.

RESULTS:

- the mean age at which children met the trial's entry criteria was 15 months

- 82% of children in the early placement group received ear tubes by the age of 3 years, while 64% received ear tubes within 60 days of randomization

181 McCarthy D. Manual for the McCarthy Scales of Children's Abilities. San Antonio, Tex.: Psychological Corporation, 1972.

182 Dunn LM and Dunn LM. Peabody Picture Vocabulary Test – Revised: manual for forms L and M. Circle Pines, Minn.: American Guidance Service, 1981.

183 Abidin RR. Parenting Stress Index: professional manual. 3rd ed. Odessa, Fla.: Psychological Assessment Resources, 1995.

184 Achenbach TM. Manual for the Child Behavior Checklist/2-3 and 1992 profile. Burlington: University of Vermont Department of Psychiatry, 1992.

- 34% of children in the delayed placement group received ear tubes by the age of 3 years, while 4% received ear tubes within 60 days of randomization

Table 1: Summary of the Trial's Key Findings

Outcome	Early Placement Group	Delayed Placement Group	P Value
Percentage of children with ear effusion >50% of days during the first 12 months of trial	14%	45%	<0.001
Mean percentage of days with ear effusion			
during first 12 months	29%	48%	<0.001
during first 24 months	30%	40%	<0.001
Mean General Cognitive Index Score[a]	99	101	Non-significant[c]
Mean Receptive Language Score[a]	92	92	Non-significant[c]
Mean Number of Different Words[a]	124	126	Non-significant[c]
Mean Parental Stress Index[b]	66	68	Non-significant[c]
Mean Child Behavior Checklist Score[b]	50	49	Non-significant[c]

[a]Higher scores signify more favorable results.
[b]Lower scores signify more favorable results.
[c]P values not reported.

Criticisms and Limitations: Children in the delayed placement group had a higher rate of persistent ear effusion, which in most cases was accompanied by conductive hearing loss. Even though the hearing of children in the delayed placement group was temporarily impaired, this did not affect developmental outcomes.

Other Relevant Studies and Information:

- The authors continued to follow children in this trial for several additional years, monitoring developmental outcomes including auditory processing, literacy, attention, social skills, and academic achievement. During follow-up, no difference were noted between children in the early vs. delayed tube placement groups at the ages of 4 years[185], 6 years[186], and 9-11 years[187].

- A clinical practice guideline from the American Academies of Pediatrics, Family Physicians, and Otolaryngology-Head and Neck Surgery recommends that for persistent effusion in otherwise asymptomatic children 2 months - 12 years who are not at risk of speech, language, or learning problems and who do not have "considerable" hearing loss, intervention is unnecessary even if effusion persists for >3 months. Instead, the guideline recommends that such children be reexamined at 3-6 month intervals until effusion is no longer present.[188] Previous guidelines, issued prior to publication of this trial by the U.S. Agency for Health Care Policy and Research, recommended ear tube placement for effusion lasting 4-6 months in all children 1-3 years with any degree of bilateral hearing loss[189].

- Studies have suggested that ear tubes are frequently placed in children unnecessarily[190].

SUMMARY AND IMPLICATIONS:

Although children with otitis media and persistent ear effusion who received early ear tube placement had lower rates of persistent effusion than did children who received delayed or no tube placement, developmental outcomes were no different in the two groups. In addition, children in the delayed placement group underwent considerably fewer ear tube procedures.

---

185 Paradise et al. Otitis media and tympanostomy tube insertion during the first three years of life: developmental outcomes at the age of four years. Pediatrics. 2003;112:265-277.

186 Paradise et al. Developmental outcomes after early or delayed insertion of tympanostomy tubes. N Engl J Med. 2005;353:576-586.

187 Paradise et al. Tympanostomy tubes and developmental outcomes at 9 to 11 years of age. N Engl J Med. 2007 Jan 18;356(3):248-261.

188 American Academy of Family Physicians; American Academy of Otolaryngology-Head and Neck Surgery; American Academy of Pediatrics Subcommittee on Otitis Media With Effusion. Otitis media with effusion. Pediatrics. 2004 May;113(5):1412-29.

189 Stool et al. Otitis media with effusion in young children. Clinical Practice Guideline, no. 12. Rockville, MD: Agency for Health Care Policy and Research, July 1994. (AHCPR publication no. 94-0622).

190 Keyhani et al. Overuse of tympanostomy tubes in New York metropolitan area: evidence from five hospital cohort. BMJ. 2008 Oct 3;337:a1607.doi:10.1136/bmj.a1607.

CLINICAL CASE: EAR TUBE PLACEMENT IN CHILDREN WITH PERSISTENT OTITIS MEDIA

CASE HISTORY:

A two year old boy is brought to your office by his parents three months after he was treated for acute otitis media. He also was treated for acute otitis media at the age of one year. The boy is doing much better now, and has achieved all of his developmental milestones including language acquisition. On examination of his ears, you note that the tympanic membrane of the affected ear is no longer red or bulging, however he has a bilateral effusion.

Based on the results of this trial, how should you treat his effusion?

SUGGESTED ANSWER:

This trial found that early placement of ear tubes did not lead to improved developmental outcomes. Since the boy in this vignette is similar to the children included in this trial and is apparently asymptomatic, he should be observed for at least several additional months before considering ear tube placement. If the effusion persists for a longer period, or if he develops learning difficulties, substantial hearing loss, or repeated episodes of acute middle ear infection, ear tube placement should be considered.

INHALED CORTICOSTEROIDS FOR MILD PERSISTENT ASTHMA:

THE START TRIAL[191]

"Our study has shown that once-daily, low-dose budesonide decreases the risk of severe [asthma] exacerbations ... in patients with mild persistent asthma. The benefits of this treatment outweigh the small effect on growth in children."

- Pauwels et al.[191]

Research Question: Do inhaled corticosteroids improve outcomes in patients with recent onset mild persistent asthma?

Funding: The AstraZeneca pharmaceutical company.

Year Study Began: 1996

Year Study Published: 2003

Study Location: 499 sites in 32 countries

191 Pauwels et al. Early intervention with budesonide in mild persistent asthma: a randomized, double-blind trial. Lancet. 2003 Mar 29;361:1071-1076.

Who Was Studied: Patients 5 to 66 years old with mild persistent asthma defined as "wheeze, cough, dyspnea, or chest tightening at least once per week, but not as often as daily." Patients were also required to have evidence of reversible airway obstruction on pulmonary function tests (an increase in the FEV_1 ≥12% after bronchodilator administration, a decrease in the FEV_1 ≥15% with exercise, or a variation of ≥15% "between the two highest and two lowest peak expiratory flow rates during 14 days").

Table 1: Asthma Classification in Adults and Children ≥5[a]

Classification	Days Per Week with Symptoms	Nights Per Month with Symptoms
Intermittent	≤2	≤2
Mild Persistent[b]	>2	3-4
Moderate Persistent	daily	≥5
Severe Persistent	continuous	frequent

[a]From the National Asthma Education and Prevention Program guidelines.
[b]Most patients in START would be classified as having mild persistent asthma.

Who Was Excluded: Patients with symptoms of asthma for >2 years, those with a history of corticosteroid treatment for more than 30 days, those whose physician felt that corticosteroids should be initiated immediately, those with a pre-bronchodilator FEV_1 <60% predicted or a post-bronchodilator FEV_1 <80% predicted, and those with "another clinically significant disease."

How Many Patients: 7,241

Study Overview:

Figure 1: Summary of START's Design

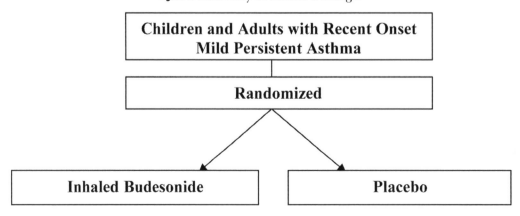

Study Intervention: Patients 11 years of age and older in the inhaled budesonide group received a dose of 400 µg once daily while those under 11 received a dose of 200 µg once daily. Patients in the placebo group received an inhaled lactose placebo.

Patients in both groups received additional asthma medications, such as inhaled bronchodilators, at the discretion of their physicians. Physicians could prescribe all approved asthma medications including both inhaled and systemic steroids.

Follow-Up: 3 years

Endpoints: Primary outcome: the time to first severe asthma-related event (an event requiring "admission or emergency treatment for worsening asthma or death due to asthma"). Secondary outcomes: proportion of symptom-free days (based on symptom notebooks kept by patients); the need for additional asthma medications; and the change in pre-bronchodilator and post-bronchodilator FEV_1.

RESULTS:

- the mean age of study participants was 24, and 55% were under 18

- the mean pre-bronchodilator response of study participants at baseline was 86% predicted and the mean post-bronchodilator response was 96% predicted

- 23.6% of patients in the placebo group were taking inhaled corticosteroids at the end of the study (recall that in both groups additional asthma medications, including corticosteroids, could be prescribed by each patient's physician for uncontrolled symptoms)

- children ages 5-15 in the budesonide group grew an average of 0.43 cm less per year than children in the control group

Table 2: Summary of START's Key Findings

Outcome	Budesonide Group	Placebo Group	P Value
Patients with at least one severe asthma-related event[a]	3.5%	6.5%	<0.0001
Proportion of symptom-free days[a]	89%	91%	<0.0001
Patients receiving at least one course of systemic steroids	15%	23%	<0.0001
Change in percent predicted prebronchodilator FEV_1	+3.49%	+1.77%	<0.0001
Change in percent predicted post-bronchodilator FEV_1	-1.79%	-2.68%	0.0005

[a]Exact percentages are not reported. These numbers are approximate values from figures.

Criticisms and Limitations: The study does not address how inhaled budesonide compares with other inhaled corticosteroids for the treatment of asthma, nor does it provide information about the optimal dose or dosing strategy for inhaled corticosteroids.

Other Relevant Studies and Information:

- At the completion of the START trial, all patients – both those in the placebo and budesonide groups – were treated with two additional years of open-label budesonide. After a total of five years of follow-up, patients in the budesonide group continued to have fewer severe asthma-related events and to require fewer additional asthma medications[192]. Additional analyses of the START trial data have also suggested that budesonide treatment is cost effective[193,194].

---

192 Busse et al. The Inhaled Steroid Treatment As Regular Therapy in Early Asthma (START) study 5-year follow-up: effectiveness of early intervention with budesonide in mild persistent asthma. J Allergy Clin Immunol. 2008;121(5):1167.

193 Sullivan et al. Cost-effectiveness analysis of early intervention with budesonide in mild persistent asthma. J Allergy Clin Immunol. 2003 Dec;122(6):1229-36.

194 Weiss et al. Cost-effectiveness analysis of early intervention with once-daily budesonide in children with mild persistent asthma: results from the START study. Pediatr Allergy Immunol. 2006 May;17 Suppl 17:21-7.

- Several other studies have also demonstrated the benefit of inhaled corticosteroids in patients with asthma[195,196].

- The START trial demonstrated a small reduction in height with budesonide, however another analysis suggested that children with asthma who receive long-term treatment with budesonide attain a normal adult height[197].

- A trial involving preschool children with recurrent wheezing compared daily budesonide vs. an intermittent use strategy in which children were treated only during episodes of respiratory tract infections. Children in both groups had similar outcomes, however children in the intermittent dosing group required less medication[198]. Other studies comparing intermittent use of inhaled corticosteroids vs. daily use have come to similar conclusions[199].

SUMMARY AND IMPLICATIONS:

The START trial showed that daily inhaled budesonide reduces severe asthma exacerbations in children and adults with recent onset mild persistent asthma. Children 5-15 treated with budesonide had a small but detectable reduction in height compared to children treated with placebo during the three year study period. Inhaled corticosteroids are the recommended first-line controller medication for both children and adults with persistent asthma.

---

195 Adams et al. Fluticasone vs. placebo for chronic asthma in adults and children. Cochrane Database Syst Rev. 2005.

196 Adams et al. Budesonide for chronic asthma in children and adults. Cochrane Database Syst Rev. 2001.

197 Agertoft and Pederson. Effect of long-term treatment with inhaled budesonide on adult height in children with asthma. N Engl J Med. 2000 Oct 12;343(15):1064-9.

198 Zeiger et al. Daily or intermittent budesonide in preschool children with recurrent wheezing. N Engl J Med. 2011 Nov 24;365(21):1990-2001.

199 Papi et al. Rescue use of beclomethasone and albuterol in a single inhaler for mild asthma. N Engl J Med. 2007 May 17;356(20):2040-52.

CLINICAL CASE: INHALED CORTICOSTEROIDS FOR MILD PERSISTENT ASTHMA

CASE HISTORY:

An 8 year-old boy with mild asthma since childhood visits your clinic because his asthma has gotten worse over the past month. Instead of using his albuterol inhaler only occasionally, he has recently been using it 3-4 times per week. In addition, he has woken up during the night three times in the past month due to his asthma. Upon further questioning, you discover that the boy's parents have been doing construction in their garage over the past month, and their house has been particularly dusty.

Based on the START trial, how should you treat this boy's asthma?

SUGGESTED ANSWER:

The START trial showed that daily inhaled budesonide reduces severe asthma exacerbations in children and adults with mild persistent asthma. Over the past month, the boy in this vignette has required albuterol more than twice a week and has had 3 nocturnal awakenings per month due to asthma. If these symptoms were to be sustained, this boy would appropriately be classified as having mild persistent asthma.

However, the worsening of this boy's asthma is likely attributable to the dust in his house. You should explain to his parents that the construction in their garage is likely worsening his symptoms, and they should identify ways to reduce their son's exposure to the dust. While it would not be unreasonable to prescribe an inhaled corticosteroid for this boy until the construction is complete, he should not be continued on the steroid indefinitely since such treatment is likely unnecessary and there are adverse effects (e.g. a small but detectable reduction in height, at least in the short term).

THE MULTIMODAL TREATMENT STUDY OF CHILDREN WITH ATTENTION-DEFICIT/ HYPERACTIVITY DISORDER (MTA)[200]

"For ADHD symptoms, our carefully crafted medication management was superior to behavioral treatment and to routine community care ..."

- The MTA Cooperative Group[200]

Research Question: What is the most effective management strategy in children with Attention-Deficit/Hyperactivity Disorder (ADHD): 1) medication management; 2) behavioral treatment; 3) a combination of medication management and behavioral treatment; or 4) routine community care?

Funding: The National Institute of Mental Health and the Department of Education.

200 The MTA Cooperative Group. A 14-month randomized clinical trial of treatment strategies for attention-deficit/hyperactivity disorder. Arch Gen Psychiatry. 1999;56:1073-1086.

Year Study Began: 1992

Year Study Published: 1999

Study Location: 8 clinical research sites in the U.S. and Canada

Who Was Studied: Children between the ages of 7 and 9.9 years meeting DSM-IV criteria for ADHD Combined Type (the most common type of ADHD in which children have symptoms of both hyperactivity and inattention). The diagnosis of ADHD was confirmed by study researchers based on parental reports and, for borderline cases, teacher reports. Children were recruited from mental health facilities, pediatricians, advertisements, and from school notices.

Who Was Excluded: Children who could not fully participate in assessments and/or treatments.

How Many Patients: 579

Study Overview:

Figure 1: Summary of MTA's Design

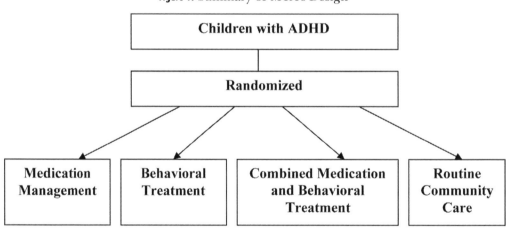

Study Intervention: *Arm 1: Medication Management-* Children in this group first received 28 days of methylphenidate at various doses to determine the appropriate dose (based on parent and teacher ratings). Children who did not respond adequately were given alternative medications such as dextroamphetamine. Subsequently, children met monthly with a pharmacotherapist who adjusted the medications using a standardized protocol based on input from parents and teachers.

Arm 2: Behavioral Treatment- Parents and children in this group participated in "parent training, child-focused treatment, and a school-based intervention." The parent training consisted of 27 group and 8 individual sessions per family led by a doctoral-level psychotherapist. The sessions initially occurred weekly, but were tapered over time. The child-focused treatment consisted of an 8-week full-time summer program that promoted the development of social skills and appropriate classroom behavior, and involved group activities. The school-based intervention involved 10-16 individual consultation sessions with each teacher conducted by the same psychotherapist. Teachers were taught how to promote appropriate behavior in the classroom. In addition, children were assisted daily by a classroom aide working under the psychologist's supervision for 12 weeks.

Arm 3: Combined Treatment- Parents and children in this group received both medication management and behavioral treatment. Information was "regularly shared" between the counselors and the pharmacotherapists so that medication changes and behavioral treatment interventions could be coordinated.

Arm 4: Community Care- Children in this group were referred to community providers and treated according to routine standards.

Follow-Up: 14 months

Endpoints: The authors assessed six major outcome domains:

1. ADHD symptoms based on parent and teacher ratings on a standardized instrument called SNAP[201]

2. Five other outcome domains including:
   ➢ Oppositional/aggressive symptoms based on parent and teacher SNAP ratings
   ➢ Social skills based on parent and teacher ratings on the standardized Social Skills Rating System (SSRS)[202]
   ➢ Internalizing symptoms (anxiety and depression) based on parent and teacher ratings on the SSRS as well as children's own ratings on the Multidimensional Anxiety Scale for Children[203]

---

201 Swanson JM. School-based Assessments and Interventions for ADD Students. Irvine, Calif: KC Publications; 1992.

202 Gresham FM and Elliott SN. Social Skills Rating System: Automated System for Scoring and Interpreting Standardized Test [computer program]. Version 1. Circle Pines, Minn: American Guidance Systems; 1989.

203 March et al. The Multidimensional Anxiety Scale for Children (MASC): factor structure, reliability, and validity. J Am Acad Child Adolesc Psychiatry. 1997;36:554-565.

➤ Parent-child relations based on a parent-child relationship questionnaire
➤ Academic achievement based on reading, math, and spelling scores on the Wechsler Individual Achievement Test[204]

RESULTS:

- at the end of the study period, 87% of children in the medication management and combined treatment groups were receiving medications, and of these children 84% were receiving methylphenidate while 12% were receiving dextroamphetamine

- 49.8% of children receiving medications experienced mild side effects, 11.4% experienced moderate side effects, and 2.9% experienced severe side effects (based on parental report)

- 67.4% of children in the community care group received medications at some point during the study

- ADHD symptoms improved considerably among children in all four arms during the study period, however as noted below children receiving medication management and combined treatment had the best outcomes

SUMMARY OF MTA'S KEY FINDINGS

Medication Management vs. Behavioral Treatment

- Medication management was superior with respect to parent and teacher ratings of inattention and teacher ratings of hyperactivity/impulsivity.

Combined Treatment vs. Medication Management

- There were no significant differences for any of the primary outcome domains. In secondary analyses of global outcomes, however, combined treatment offered slight advantages over medication management alone, particularly among children with complex presentations of ADHD.

---

204 Wechsler Individual Achievement Test: Manual. San Antionio, Tex: Psychological Corp; 1992.

- Children in the combined treatment group also required lower average daily medication doses than those in the medication management group (31.2 mg vs. 37.7 mg)

Combined Treatment vs. Behavioral Treatment

- Combined treatment was superior with respect to parent and teacher ratings of inattention and parent ratings of hyperactivity/impulsivity, parent ratings of oppositional/aggressive symptoms, and reading scores.

Community Care vs. Other Study Treatments

- Medication management and combined treatment were generally superior to community care for ADHD symptoms and for some of the other outcome domains.

- Behavioral treatment and community care were similar for ADHD symptoms, however behavioral treatment was superior to community care for parent-child relations.

Criticisms and Limitations: While the MTA trial demonstrated the superiority of a particular medication management strategy vs. a particular behavioral treatment strategy, medication management may not always be superior to behavioral treatment, i.e. it is possible that a different behavioral treatment strategy might be equivalent or even superior to medication management.

The medication management and behavioral treatment strategies used in this trial were time-intensive and might not be practical in some real-world settings.

Other Relevant Studies and Information: After the MTA trial was completed, study children returned to their usual community care team for ongoing treatment. A three-year follow-up analysis (22 months after the trial was concluded and children returned to usual community care) demonstrated the following:

- the percentage of children taking regular ADHD medications increased in the behavioral treatment group to 45%

- the percentage of children taking regular ADHD medications decreased in the medication management and combined treatment groups to 71%

- the percentage of children taking regular ADHD medications remained relatively constant in the community care group at 62%

- symptoms after three years were no different among the treatment groups for any measure, i.e. the initial advantage of medication management and combined treatment was no longer apparent

Guidelines from the American Academy of Pediatrics for children with ADHD recommend[205]:

- medications and/or behavioral treatment for children <12 depending on family preference
- medications with or without behavioral therapy as first-line treatment for children 12-18 (behavioral therapy can be used instead if the child and family do not want medications)

SUMMARY AND IMPLICATIONS:

For children with ADHD, carefully controlled medication management was superior to behavioral treatment and to routine community care during the 14-month study period. This benefit did not persist three years after randomization (after children had returned to usual community care). Children receiving combined medication and behavioral treatment had similar outcomes as those receiving medications alone, however these children required lower medication doses to control their symptoms. Despite its limitations, the MTA trial is frequently cited as evidence that carefully controlled medications are superior to behavioral treatment for children with ADHD. Nevertheless, behavioral therapy may be an appropriate and efficacious first-line therapy for some children <12 when the child and family prefer this approach.

CLINICAL CASE: MANAGEMENT OF ADHD

CASE HISTORY:

A 6 year old boy is diagnosed with ADHD based on reports from his teachers and parents that he has a short attention span and is hyperactive, sometimes disrupting classroom activities. His school performance has been adequate,

---

205 ADHD: Clinical Practice Guideline for the Diagnosis, Evaluation, and Treatment of Attention-Deficit/ Hyperactivity Disorder in Children and Adolescents. American Academy of Pediatrics. Pediatrics. October 16, 2011.

however both his teachers and parents believe he would perform better if his attention span improved.

Based on the results of the MTA trial, should this boy be treated for his ADHD with medications, behavioral therapy, or both?

SUGGESTED ANSWER:

The MTA trial suggests that symptoms of ADHD are better controlled with medications than with behavioral therapy. Still, because medications may have adverse effects, the American Academy of Pediatrics recommends either medications, behavioral therapy, or both as first-line treatment for ADHD in children <12. Therefore, the boy in this vignette could initially be treated with either approach based on the preference of the family.

MEASLES, MUMPS, AND RUBELLA VACCINATION AND AUTISM[206]

"This study provides strong evidence against the hypothesis that MMR vaccination causes autism."

- Madsen et al.[206]

Research Question: Does the Measles, Mumps, and Rubella vaccine (MMR) cause autism?

Funding: The Danish National Research Foundation, the Centers for Disease Control and Prevention, and the National Alliance for Autism Research.

Year Study Began: data from 1991 – 1999 were included (the data were collected retrospectively)

Year Study Published: 2002

Study Location: Denmark

206 Madsen et al. A population-based study of measles, mumps, and rubella vaccination and autism. NEJM. 2002 Nov 347;19: 1477-1482.

Who Was Studied: All children born in Denmark between January 1991 and December 1998 (all Danish children are entered into a national registry at birth).

Who Was Excluded: Children with tuberous sclerosis, Angelman's syndrome, fragile X syndrome, and congenital rubella – all of which are associated with autism.

How Many Patients: 537,303 children, 82% of whom received the MMR vaccine and 18% of whom did not.

Study Overview: The rates of autism among children who received the MMR vaccine were compared to the rates among those who did not.

Figure 1: Summary of the Study's Design

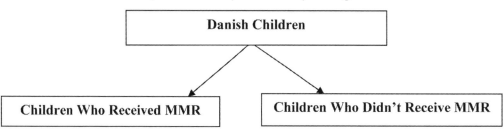

The authors used data from the Danish National Board of Health to determine which children received the MMR vaccine as well as the age of vaccine administration. The national vaccination program in Denmark recommends that children receive the MMR vaccine at 15 months of age followed by a booster at the age of 12 years.

Children were identified as having autism, as well as other autistic-spectrum disorders, using data from a national psychiatric registry (in Denmark, all patients with suspected autism are referred to child psychiatrists, and when a diagnosis of autism is made it is entered into the registry). The authors also recorded the date when the diagnosis was made, allowing them to determine the time interval between vaccine administration and autism diagnosis.

The authors controlled for differences between vaccinated and unvaccinated children. They did this by adjusting for factors such as age, sex, socioeconomic status, mother's education level, and the child's gestational age at birth.

Follow-Up: Children were monitored for autism from the time they reached one year of age until the end of the study period (December 31, 1999). The mean age of children at the end of the study period was approximately 5 years.

Endpoints: Rates of autism and rates of autistic-spectrum disorders.

RESULTS:

- 82% of children in the study received the MMR vaccine, and the mean age of vaccination was 17 months

- among children diagnosed with autism, the mean age of diagnosis was 4 years and 3 months

- the prevalence of autism among eight-year-olds in the study was 7.7 per 10,000 (0.08%), which was consistent with rates from other countries at the time

Table 1: Summary of the Study's Key Findings

Outcomes	Adjusted Relative Risk of Autism Among Vaccinated vs. Unvaccinated Children[a] (95% Confidence Intervals)
Autism	0.92 (0.68-1.24)
Autistic-Spectrum Disorders	0.83 (0.65-1.07)

[a]A relative risk <1.0 means a lower rate of autism among vaccinated children compared with unvaccinated children.

- there was no clustering of autism diagnoses at any time interval after vaccination, nor was there an association between the age at which the vaccine was given and the subsequent development of autism (arguing against a link between vaccination and the development of autism)

Criticisms and Limitations: The authors attempted to control for differences between vaccinated and unvaccinated children. However, since this was not a randomized trial, it is possible that the authors did not control for all potential confounders. For example, parents of children with a family history of autism may have been more likely to withhold vaccination because of media reports warning about a link between the MMR vaccine and autism. As a result, children with a family history of autism – and presumably an increased risk – may have disproportionately opted not to be vaccinated, potentially masking an increased rate of autism due to the vaccine.

In addition, although the authors did not identify a clustering of autism diagnoses at various time intervals following vaccination, the dataset did not contain the date when the first symptoms of autism were noted. Thus, it is possible that there was a clustering of first autism symptoms – but not diagnoses – at certain time intervals following vaccination.

Other Relevant Studies and Information:

- Children typically begin to show signs and symptoms of autism in the second and third years of life – shortly after most guidelines recommend that children receive the MMR vaccine. This may explain why some parents (and experts) associate the vaccine with autism.

- Several other observational studies have also failed to show a link between the MMR vaccine and autism[207,208,209]. Several studies have also failed to show a link between thimerosal – a mercury-containing ingredient that used to be included in many childhood vaccines – and autism[210,211,212].

- One widely cited article[213], which was subsequently retracted by the journal that published it[214], reported on a series of children who appeared to develop GI symptoms as well as signs of autism soon after receiving the MMR vaccine. The article generated considerable media attention as well as concern among parents, however the results have widely been called into question due to concerns about falsified data.

SUMMARY AND IMPLICATIONS:

This large cohort study did not identify a link between MMR vaccination and autism or autism-spectrum disorders. In addition, there was no clustering

207 Taylor et al. Autism and measles, mumps, and rubella vaccine: no epidemiological evidence for a causal association. Lancet. 1999;353(9169):2026-9.

208 Mrozek-Budzyn et al. Lack of association between measles-mumps-rubella vaccination and autism in children: a case-control study. Pediatr Infect Dis J. 2010;29(5):397-400.

209 Smeeth et al. MMR vaccination and pervasive developmental disorders: a case-control study. Lancet. 2004;364(9438):963-9.

210 Madsen et al. Thimerosal and the occurrence of autism: negative ecological evidence from Danish population-based data. Pediatrics. 2003;112(3 Pt 1):604-6.

211 Hviid et al. Association between thimerosal-containing vaccine and autism. JAMA. 2003;290(13):1763-6.

212 Thompson et al. Early thimerosal exposure and neuropsychological outcomes at 7 to 10 years. N Engl J Med. 2007;357(13):1281-92.

213 Wakefield et al. Ileal-lymphoid-nodular hyperplasia, non-specific colitis, and pervasive developmental disorder in children. Lancet. 1998;351(9103):637-41.

214 Retraction–Ileal-lymphoid-nodular hyperplasia, non-specific colitis, and pervasive developmental disorder in children. Lancet. 2010;375(9713):445.

of autism diagnoses at any time interval after vaccination. These findings argue against a link between vaccination and the development of autism.

CLINICAL CASE: MEASLES, MUMPS, AND RUBELLA VACCINATION AND AUTISM

CASE HISTORY:

Nervous parents bring their 15-month old baby girl to your office. Their previous pediatrician suggested that they find a new doctor after they declined MMR vaccination for their daughter. The girl's mother is concerned about the MMR vaccine because her nephew developed symptoms of autism shortly after he was vaccinated. The parents want your perspective on the vaccine. Do the data support a link between MMR vaccination and autism? Will you care for their child if they decline vaccination?

SUGGESTED ANSWER:

This study, as well as several others, have failed to show a link between MMR vaccination and autism. In addition, the most widely cited analysis suggesting a link between MMR vaccination and autism has been called into question due to concerns about falsified data. Although none of these studies has conclusively ruled out a very small link between MMR vaccination and autism, the preponderance of evidence suggests that there is not.

One way to respond to these parents would be to explain that numerous studies of high methodological quality have failed to demonstrate a link between the MMR vaccine and autism. While it is impossible to entirely exclude a very small association, it is likely that there is not. You should also emphasize to the parents that there are clear and proven benefits of the vaccine, and that major professional organizations such as the American Academy of Pediatrics strongly recommend vaccination for all children. If the parents remain concerned, they might consider delaying vaccination for several months until the child is older.

If the parents opt not to have their daughter vaccinated, you will need to decide whether to continue caring for their child. Most physicians will care for unvaccinated children while continuing to encourage vaccination, however a small percentage choose not to.

SECTION 6:

RADIOLOGY

MAGNETIC RESONANCE IMAGING FOR LOW BACK PAIN[215]

"Although ... patients preferred [rapid MRI scans to plain radiographs for the evaluation of low back pain], substituting rapid MRI for radiographic evaluations ... may offer little additional benefit to patients, and it may increase the costs of care because of the increased number of spine operations that patients are likely to undergo."

- Jarvik et al.[215]

Research Question: Should patients with low back pain requiring imaging be offered plain radiographs or magnetic resonance imaging (MRI)?

Funding: The Agency for Healthcare Research and Quality and the National Institute for Arthritis and Musculoskeletal and Skin Diseases.

Year Study Began: 1998

---

215 Jarvik et al. Rapid magnetic resonance imaging vs radiographs for patients with low back pain: a randomized controlled trial. JAMA. 2003;289(21):2810-2718.

Year Study Published: 2003

Study Location: 4 imaging sites in Washington State (an outpatient clinic, a teaching hospital; a multispecialty clinic, and a private imaging center)

Who Was Studied: Adults 18 years and older referred by their physician for radiographs of the lumbar spine to evaluate lower back pain and/or radiculopathy.

Who Was Excluded: Patients with lumbar surgery within the previous year, those with acute external trauma, and those with metallic implants in the spine.

How Many Patients: 380

Study Overview:

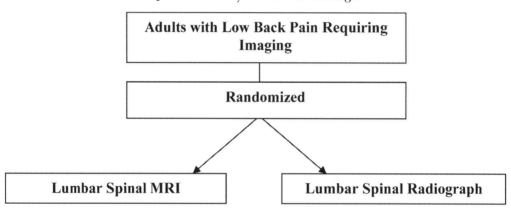

Figure 1: Summary of the Trial's Design

Study Intervention: Patients assigned to the plain radiograph group received the films according to standard protocol. Most patients received anteroposterior and lateral views only, however a small number received additional views when requested by the ordering physician.

Patients assigned to the MRI group were scheduled for the scan on the day of study enrollment whenever possible, and if not within a week of enrollment. Most scans were performed with a field strength of 1.5 T, and all patients received sagittal and axial T2-weighted images.

Follow-Up: 12 months

Endpoints: Primary outcome: Scores on the 23-item modified Roland-Morris back pain disability scale[216]. Secondary outcomes: quality of life as assessed

---

216 Roland M and Morris R. A study of the natural history of back pain, 1: development of a reliable and sensitive measure of disability in low back pain. Spine. 1983;8:141-144.

using the Medical Outcomes Study 36-Item Short Form Survey (SF-36)[217]; patient satisfaction with care as assessed using the Deyo-Diehl patient satisfaction questionnaire[218]; days of lost work; patient reassurance; and health care resource utilization.

The 23-item modified Roland-Morris back pain disability scale consists of 23 'yes' or 'no' questions. Patients are given one point for each 'yes' answer for a total possible score of 23. Below are sample questions on the scale:

- I stay at home most of the time because of my back problem or leg pain (sciatica)

- I walk more slowly than usual because of my back problem or leg pain (sciatica)

- I stay in bed most of the time because of my back or leg pain (sciatica)

RESULTS:

- the mean age of study patients was 53, 15% were either unemployed, disabled, or on leave from work, 24% had depression, and 70% reported pain radiating to the legs

- 49% of patients were referred for imaging by primary care doctors while 51% were referred by specialists

- the spinal MRI revealed disk herniation in 33% of patients, nerve root impingement in 7%, moderate or severe central canal stenosis in 20%, and lateral recess stenosis in 17% – findings that are typically not detectable with plain radiographs

---

217 Ware JE and Sherbourne CD. The MOS 36-item short-form survey (SF-36), I: conceptual framework and item selection. Med Care. 1992;30:473-483.

218 Deyo RA and Diehl AK. Patient satisfaction with medical care for low-back pain. Spine. 1986;11:28-30.

Table 1: The Trial's Key Findings After 12 Months[a]

Outcome	Radiograph Group	MRI Group	P Value
Roland-Morris Back Pain Score (Scale: 0-23)[b]	8.75	9.34	0.53
SF-36, Physical Functioning (Scale: 0-100)[c]	63.77	61.04	not significant[d]
Patient Satisfaction (Scale: 0-11)[c]	7.34	7.04	not significant[d]
Days of Lost Work in Past 4 Weeks	1.26	1.57	not significant[d]
Were you reassured by the imaging results?	58%	74%	0.002

[a]The 12-month outcomes were adjusted for baseline scores, e.g. the 12-month Roland scores were adjusted for the fact that, at baseline, scores were slightly higher in patients randomized to the MRI group.
[b]Higher scores indicate a worse outcome.
[c]Higher scores indicate a better outcome.
[d]Actual P value not reported.

Table 2: Comparison of Resource Utilization During the Study Period

Outcome	Radiograph Group	MRI Group	P Value
Patients Receiving Opioid Analgesics	25%	26%	0.94
Subsequent MRIs Per Patient	0.22	0.09	0.01
Physical Therapy, Acupuncture, and Massage Visits Per Patient	7.9	3.8	0.008
Specialist Consultations Per Patient	0.49	0.73	0.07
Patients Receiving Lumbar Spine Surgery	2%	6%	0.09
Total Costs of Health Care Services	$1,651	$2,121	0.11

Criticisms and Limitations: The increased rate of spinal surgeries and the higher cost of health care services in the MRI group did not reach statistical significance. Therefore, it is not appropriate to draw firm conclusions from these findings.

Other Relevant Studies and Information:

- Other trials have suggested that early spinal imaging (radiographs, computed tomography, and MRI) does not improve outcomes in patients with acute lower back pain without alarm symptoms such as worsening neurologic function[219], nor does it substantially assist with decision making in patients referred for epidural steroid injections of the spine[220]

- Guidelines[221] recommend that MRIs of the lumbar spine only be obtained in patients with signs or symptoms of:

  - ➢ emergent conditions such as the cauda equina syndrome, tumors, infections, or fractures with neurologic impingement
  - ➢ radicular symptoms severe enough and long-lasting enough to warrant surgical intervention
  - ➢ spinal stenosis severe enough and long-lasting enough to warrant surgical intervention

SUMMARY AND IMPLICATIONS:

Although spinal MRIs (compared with plain radiographs) are reassuring for patients with low back pain, they do not lead to improved functional outcomes. In addition, spinal MRIs detect anatomical abnormalities that would otherwise go undiscovered, possibly leading to spinal surgeries of uncertain value.

---

219 Chou et al. Imaging strategies for low-back pain: systematic review and meta-analysis. Lancet. 2009;373(9662):463.

220 Cohen et al. Effect of MRI on Treatment Results or Decision Making in Patients With Lumbosacral Radiculopathy Referred for Epidural Steroid Injections: A Multicenter, Randomized Controlled Trial. Arch Intern Med. 2011 Dec 12.

221 Bigos, SJ, Bowyer, OR, Braen, GR, et al. Acute low back pain problems in adults. Clinical practice guideline No 14. Agency for Health Care Policy and Research, Public Health Service, US Department of Health and Human Services, Rockville, MD, December 1994.

CLINICAL CASE: MRI FOR LOW BACK PAIN

CASE HISTORY:

A 52 year old man with 6 weeks of low back pain visits your office requesting an MRI of his spine. His symptoms began after doing yard work and have improved only slightly during this time period. The pain is bothersome, but not incapacitating, and radiates down his right leg. He has no systemic symptoms (fevers, chills, or weight loss) and denies bowel or bladder dysfunction. He reports difficulty walking due to the pain. On exam, he is an overweight man in no apparent distress. His range of motion is limited due to pain. He has no neurological deficits.

Based on the results of this trial, should you order an MRI for this patient?

SUGGESTED ANSWER:

Based on the results of this trial, ordering a spinal MRI in a patient like the one in this vignette is unlikely to lead to improved functional outcomes and may increase the likelihood of spinal surgery by detecting anatomical abnormalities that would otherwise go undiscovered. Still, this trial showed that an MRI may provide reassurance to patients. For this reason, you should reassure your patient in other ways, for example by telling him that he does not have any signs or symptoms of a serious back problem like an infection or cancer.

Other types of spinal imaging such as plain radiographs do not appear to improve outcomes in patients with acute low back pain without alarm symptoms either. Thus, even a plain film may not be necessary at this time.

SCREENING FOR CORONARY ARTERY DISEASE IN ASYMPTOMATIC PATIENTS WITH DIABETES:

THE DIAD STUDY[222]

"The strategy of routine screening for [coronary artery disease] in patients with type 2 diabetes is based on the premise that testing could accurately identify a significant number of individuals at particularly high risk and lead to various interventions that prevent cardiac events. However, the results of the DIAD study would appear to refute this notion."

- Young et al.[222]

---

222 Young et al. Cardiac outcomes after screening for asymptomatic coronary artery disease in patients with type 2 diabetes: the DIAD study: a randomized controlled trial. JAMA. 2009 Apr 15;301(15):1547-55.

Research Question: Should asymptomatic patients with type 2 diabetes – who are at high risk for cardiac events – be screened for coronary artery disease (CAD)?

Funding: The National Institutes of Health, Bristol Myers-Squibb Medical Imaging, and Astellas Pharma.

Year Study Began: 2000

Year Study Published: 2009

Study Location: 14 centers in the U.S. and Canada

Who Was Studied: Adults 50-75 years of age with type 2 diabetes.

Who Was Excluded: Patients with symptoms of angina, recent stress testing or coronary angiography, prior cardiac events, a markedly abnormal baseline electrocardiogram, or a limited life expectancy.

How Many Patients: 1,123

Study Overview:

Figure 1: Summary of DIAD's Design

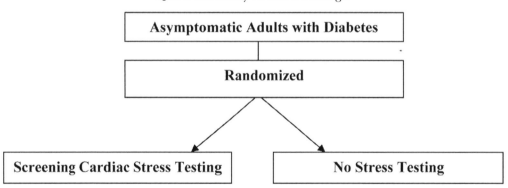

Study Intervention: Patients in the group assigned to cardiac stress testing received an adenosine-stress and radionuclide myocardial perfusion scan. Those with abnormal stress tests were managed according to the judgment of their providers (i.e. they might be managed with medical therapy or they might receive follow-up coronary angiography and/or revascularization at their physician's discretion). Patients in the control group did not undergo stress testing unless they developed symptoms for which stress testing was indicated.

Follow-Up: Mean 4.8 years

Endpoints: Primary outcome: a composite of nonfatal myocardial infarction and cardiac death. Secondary outcomes: unstable angina, heart failure, stroke, and coronary revascularization.

RESULTS:

- in the screening group, 22% of patients had abnormal stress tests, including 10% who had a small perfusion defect, 6% who had a moderate or large perfusion defect, and 6% who had a non-perfusion abnormality

- 2% of patients with normal test results and 2% with small perfusion defects had cardiac events during the study period compared with 12.1% of patients with moderate or large perfusion defects and 6.7% with non-perfusion abnormalities

- in the screening group, 4.4% of patients received coronary angiography within 120 days of their stress test; in comparison, 0.5% of patients in the non-screened group received coronary angiography within 120 days of randomization

Table 1: DIAD's Key Findings

Outcome	Screening Group	Non-Screened Group	P Value
Myocardial infarction or cardiac death	2.7%	3.0%	0.73
Unstable angina	0.7%	0.5%	0.70
Heart failure	1.2%	1.2%	0.99
Stroke	1.8%	0.9%	0.20
Revascularizations	5.5%	7.8%	0.14
All Cause Mortality[a]	3.2%	2.7%	0.60

[a]All cause mortality was not a predefined endpoint.

Criticisms and Limitations: Cardiac event rates in the study were lower than among the general population of patients with diabetes, perhaps because (as the authors assert) the patients were well managed with aspirin, statins, and ACE inhibitors. It is possible that screening stress tests might be beneficial among a less well managed cohort of patients. In addition, because the event rate was lower than expected, the trial was underpowered to detect small differences between the groups.

SUMMARY AND IMPLICATIONS:

Screening stress tests in patients with type 2 diabetes are abnormal 22% of the time. However, detecting these abnormalities does not appear to aid in patient management.

CLINICAL CASE: SCREENING FOR CORONARY ARTERY DISEASE IN ASYMPTOMATIC PATIENTS WITH DIABETES

CASE HISTORY:

You are evaluating a 52 year old woman with diabetes in an urgent care clinic for chest pain. The pain began three days ago after the patient spent the afternoon with her 1 year-old grandson. During that afternoon, the woman had to lift the baby numerous times. The pain occurs on the left side of her chest and back whenever she raises her arms above her head. She does not have any pain with walking, and she denies any associated symptoms such as shortness of breath, nausea, vomiting, or diaphoresis.

You believe that this woman's chest pain is musculoskeletal in origin, and that the probability of a cardiac etiology is remote. Still, the woman is at increased cardiac risk because of her diabetes, and could be having an atypical cardiac presentation. You wonder whether or not to order a stress test for this patient. Do the results of DIAD affect your thinking?

SUGGESTED ANSWER:

DIAD showed that patients with diabetes without symptoms of CAD do not appear to benefit from screening stress tests. While the woman in this vignette has chest pain, your clinical suspicion that the symptoms are due to CAD is very low. If you were to order a stress test and it was suggestive of CAD, it is likely that the chest pain she is experiencing is unrelated to the stress test findings. In order words, you probably wouldn't "believe the results" if the stress test were to be positive. Thus, ordering a stress test in this woman would likely have the same impact as ordering a stress test in an asymptomatic woman with diabetes: there would be a 22% chance that the stress test would be abnormal, however knowing this information would be unlikely to aid in the patient's treatment.

DIAGNOSING ACUTE PULMONARY EMBOLISM:

THE CHRISTOPHER STUDY[223]

"This large cohort study of ... patients with clinically suspected pulmonary embolism demonstrates that the use of [simple clinical criteria], D-dimer testing, and CT scan can guide treatment decisions ..."

- The Christopher Study Investigators[223]

Research Question: Can a simple predefined protocol involving clinical criteria (the modified Wells criteria), D-dimer testing, and computed tomography (CT) safely and effectively rule out acute pulmonary embolism (PE) among patients who are clinically suspected of this condition?

Funding: An unrestricted grant from participating hospitals.

Year Study Began: 2002

223 Christopher Study Investigators. Effectiveness of managing suspected pulmonary embolism using an algorithm combining clinical probability, D-dimer testing, and computed tomography. JAMA. 2006 Jan 11;295(2):172-9.

Year Study Published: 2006

Study Location: 12 centers in the Netherlands

Who Was Studied: Adults ≥18 with clinically suspected acute PE. Patients presenting to the emergency room (81.7%) as well as hospitalized patients (18.3%) were included. Patients were required to have "sudden onset of dyspnea, sudden deterioration of existing dyspnea, or sudden onset of pleuritic chest pain without another apparent cause."

Who Was Excluded: Patients receiving treatment doses of unfractionated or low-molecular-weight heparin for >24 hours, those with a life expectancy less than 3 months, those who were pregnant, those with an allergy to intravenous contrast, those with renal insufficiency (a creatinine clearance <30 mL/s), or those with hemodynamic instability.

How Many Patients: 3,306

Study Overview:

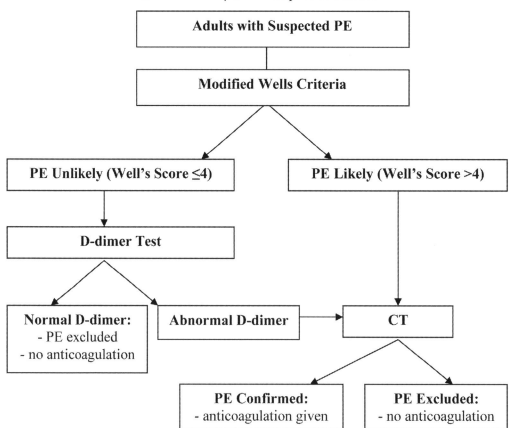

Figure 1: Summary of Christopher's Protocol

Study Intervention: Patients with a suspected PE were evaluated by an attending physician and pulmonary embolism was categorized as either "unlikely" if the modified Wells score was ≤4 or "likely" if the score was >4.

Table 1: Modified Wells Score[224]

Criteria	Points
Signs and symptoms of deep venous thrombosis (e.g. leg swelling and tenderness of deep veins)	3.0
PE more likely than alternative diagnoses	3.0
Heart rate >100 beats per minute	1.5
Immobilization for more than 3 days or surgery in previous 4 weeks	1.5
History of PE or deep venous thrombosis	1.5
Hemoptysis	1.0
Active malignancy within previous 6 months	1.0

Patients with a modified Wells score ≤4 underwent D-dimer testing, and if the test was negative (D-dimer concentration ≤500 ng/mL) the diagnosis of PE was considered excluded and anticoagulant treatment was withheld. If the D-dimer test was positive, the patient was referred for a CT angiogram of the chest. In addition, patients with a modified Wells score >4 were referred for chest CT.

When a PE was diagnosed with CT, patients received anticoagulation with unfractionated heparin or low-molecular-weight heparin followed by warfarin. When the CT did not demonstrate acute PE, anticoagulation was withheld and alternative diagnoses were considered. For inconclusive CT results (i.e. motion artifact or inadequate contrast enhancement), patients were managed according to the discretion of the attending physician.

Follow-Up: 3 months

Endpoints: Primary outcome: Symptomatic venous thromboembolic events (fatal or nonfatal PE or DVT).

---

224 Wells et al. Derivation of a simple clinical model to categorize patients' probability of pulmonary embolism: increasing the model's utility with the SimpliRED D-dimer. Thromb Haemost. 2000;83:416-420.

RESULTS:

Modified Wells Criteria and D-dimer Classifications:

- 66.7% of patients had a modified Wells score ≤4 and underwent D-dimer testing

- 52% of patients who underwent D-dimer testing had a positive result

- 68% of all patients were referred for a CT either because of an abnormal D-dimer test or because of a modified Wells score >4

CT Scan Results Among Patients Referred for CT:

- 30% of patients were found to have a PE and received anticoagulation

- 67% of patients were found not to have a PE, and anticoagulation was withheld unless there were other indications for anticoagulation

- 3% of patients had inconclusive results or did not receive the CT scan; in 10% of these situations the physician elected to start anticoagulation

Table 2: Christopher's Key Findings

Patient Groups	Nonfatal Thromboembolic Events (95% Confidence Intervals)	Fatal Thromboembolic Events (95% Confidence Intervals)
PE excluded with Well's criteria and D-dimer (32% of patients)	0.5% (0.2%-1.1%)	0% (0.0%-0.3%)
PE excluded with CT (46% of patients)	1.3% (0.7%-2.0%)	0.5% (0.2%-1.0%)
PE confirmed with CT (20% of patients)	3.0% (1.8%-4.6%)[a]	1.6% (0.8%-2.9%)[a]
CT not performed or inconclusive (2% of patients)	2.9%[b]	1.4%[b]

[a]Refers to recurrent symptomatic thromboembolic events.
[b]95% confidence intervals not reported.

Criticisms and Limitations: A high percentage of study patients (68%) ultimately required CT scans for evaluation, i.e. the protocol only prevented 32% of patients from receiving a CT.

The study did not compare alternative protocols for evaluating patients with suspected pulmonary emboli and therefore it is not known how this protocol compares with other protocols.

Other Relevant Studies and Information:

- Another study involving a different, more complicated protocol also showed the potential utility of clinical assessment, D-dimer testing, and imaging for assessing patients with suspected pulmonary emboli[225].

- The PIOPED I study showed that ventilation/perfusion lung (V/Q) scans can be helpful in confirming a PE when there is both a high clinical probability and a high radiologic suspicion for a PE. In addition, VQ scans are helping in excluding a PE when the scan is normal and when there is a low clinical probability. However, in many cases the clinical and radiologic results after V/Q scanning are contradictory and/or inconclusive[226].

- The PIOPED II study showed that CT angiography, when combined with a clinical assessment (traditional Wells criteria), accurately confirms or excludes the diagnosis of PE except when the clinical assessment and radiologic results are contradictory[227].

- The traditional Wells criteria, which use a scoring system similar to the system used in the Christopher study, categorize patients as low, intermediate, or high probability for PE[228].

SUMMARY AND IMPLICATIONS:

A simple protocol involving clinical criteria (the modified Wells criteria), D-dimer testing, and CT can safely and effectively exclude acute PE in patients who are clinically suspected of the condition. Patients who followed the protocol, which is shown in Figure 1, had very low rates of subsequent thromboembolic events after 3 months of follow-up.

---

225 Perrier et al. Multidetector-row computed tomography in suspected pulmonary embolism. NEJM. 2005; 352(17): 1760-1768.

226 The PIOPED Investigators. Value of the ventilation/perfusion scan in acute pulmonary embolism. Results of the prospective investigation of pulmonary embolism diagnosis (PIOPED). JAMA. 1990;263(20):2753-9.

227 Stein et al. Multidetector computed tomography for acute pulmonary embolism. N Engl J Med. 2006;354(22):2317-27.

228 Wells et al. Excluding pulmonary embolism at the bedside without diagnostic imaging: management of patients with suspected pulmonary embolism presenting to the emergency department by using a simple clinical model and D-dimer. Ann Intern Med 2001;135:98-107.

CLINICAL CASE: DIAGNOSING ACUTE PULMONARY EMBOLISM

CASE HISTORY:

An 85 year old man with congestive heart failure, chronic kidney disease, and a distant history of colon cancer presents to the emergency room with the relatively acute onset of worsening shortness of breath over the past 12 hours. He has had several emergency room visits and hospitalizations for heart failure exacerbations and pneumonia over the past year.

On exam, the patient has a heart rate of 110 and a respiratory rate of 24. He has elevated neck veins and bilateral lower extremity swelling.

Based on the results of the Christopher study, how should you evaluate this patient for a pulmonary embolism?

SUGGESTED ANSWER:

According to the Christopher study, patients with a suspected diagnosis of pulmonary embolism and a modified Wells score ≤4 should receive D-dimer testing to evaluate for pulmonary embolism. If the D-dimer is elevated, they should receive a chest CT to confirm or refute the diagnosis. In contrast, patients with a modified Wells score >4 should immediately receive a chest CT.

The patient in this vignette is complicated: although he presents with the sudden onset of dyspnea, an alternative diagnosis – congestive heart failure – may be a more likely cause of his symptoms. If you believe that this patient is most likely experiencing a congestive heart failure exacerbation, it would probably not be appropriate to evaluate him for a pulmonary embolism at all since only patients with clinically suspected acute pulmonary embolism were included in the Christopher study. In fact, evaluating him for a pulmonary embolism could be harmful: 68% of patients in the Christopher study ultimately underwent a CT scan, which could be damaging to his kidneys because of the contrast load.

Thus, although the Christopher study provides a helpful protocol for evaluating patients with a suspected pulmonary embolism, clinical judgment remains critical for ensuring that the protocol is used appropriately.

IDENTIFYING CHILDREN WITH LOW-RISK HEAD INJURIES WHO DO NOT REQUIRE COMPUTED TOMOGRAPHY[229]

"[We] derived and validated highly accurate prediction rules for children at very low risk of [clinically-important traumatic brain injuries] for whom CT scans should typically be avoided. Application of these rules could limit CT use, protecting children from unnecessary radiation risks."

- Kuppermann et al.[229]

Research Question: Is it possible to develop clinical prediction rules for identifying children at very low risk for clinically-important traumatic brain injuries who do not require computed tomography (CT) scans for evaluation?

---

229 Kuppermann et al. Identification of children at very low risk of clinically-important brain injuries after head trauma: a prospective cohort study. The Lancet. 2009;374:1160-1170.

Funding: The Pediatric Emergency Care Applied Research Network (PECARN), a federally funded organization supported by the United States Health Resources and Services Administration.

Year Study Began: 2004

Year Study Published: 2009

Study Location: 25 emergency departments in the U.S.

Who Was Studied: Children younger than 18 presenting to emergency departments within 24 hours of blunt traumatic head injuries.

Who Was Excluded: Children with "trivial" injuries such as ground-level falls without signs or symptoms of head injuries aside from scalp lacerations or abrasions, as well as children with penetrating trauma, brain tumors, and "pre-existing neurological disorders." In addition, children with ventricular shunts, bleeding disorders, and Glasgow Coma Scale (GCS) scores under 14 were excluded from this analysis.

How Many Patients: 42,412

Study Overview:

Figure 1: Summary of the Study's Design

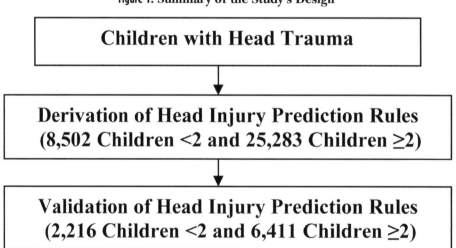

Derivation of Prediction Rules: Emergency department physicians interviewed and examined a sample of children with head trauma (the derivation sample) to collect information about each child's history and physical examination findings. This information was collected prior to head imaging (if imaging was performed). The patient information was then correlated with patient outcomes (i.e. whether or not patients were ultimately found to have clinically-important traumatic brain injuries) in order to develop prediction rules for assessing brain injury risk.

Validation of Prediction Rules: The prediction rules were then applied to a separate sample of children (the validation sample) presenting with blunt head trauma to assess how well the rules forecasted whether or not these children would ultimately be diagnosed with clinically-important traumatic brain injuries.

Determination of Patient Outcomes: Research coordinators determined which children were ultimately diagnosed with clinically-important traumatic brain injuries (ciTBI) by reviewing the medical records of all children admitted to the hospital. In addition, research coordinators conducted telephone interviews with the guardians of all children discharged from the emergency department to identify any children with missed injuries.

Clinically-important traumatic brain injuries were defined as:

- death from traumatic brain injury

- neurosurgery

- intubation for >24 hours

- hospital admission for ≥2 nights "associated with traumatic brain injury on CT"

The researchers did not classify "brief intubations" and single-night admissions for "minor CT findings" as ci-TBIs because these outcomes do not typically represent clinically-important injuries that must be identified, i.e. patient outcomes would generally be unchanged if these injuries were never diagnosed.

RESULTS:

- Table 1 lists the six predictive features for ciTBI identified using data from the derivation sample; the strongest predictors of ciTBI in both age groups were an abnormality in mental status or clinical evidence of a skull fracture

- Table 2 divides children into three risk categories using the predictive features

Table 1: Predictors of Clinically-Important Traumatic Brain Injuries

Children <2 Years	Children ≥2 Years
➢ Altered Mental Status[a]	➢ Altered Mental Status[a]
➢ Palpable or Possibly Palpable Skull Fracture	➢ Clinical Signs of Basilar Skull Fracture[c]
➢ Occipital, Parietal, or Temporal Scalp Hematoma	➢ Loss of Consciousness
➢ Loss of Consciousness ≥5 Seconds	➢ Vomiting
➢ Severe Mechanism of Injury[b]	➢ Severe Mechanism of Injury[b]
➢ Child Not Acting Normally According to Parents	➢ Severe Headache

[a]Defined as a Glasgow Coma Scale of 14 or one of the following: agitation, somnolence, repetitive questioning, or a slow response to verbal communication.
[b]Defined as motor vehicle crash with patient ejection, death of another passenger, or rollover; pedestrian or bicyclist without helmet struck by motorized vehicle; falls >5 feet for children ≥2 years or >3 feet for those <2 years; or head struck by high impact object.
[c]For example: retro-auricular bruising (Battle's sign), periorbital bruising (raccoon eyes), hematotympanum, or cerebral spinal fluid otorrhea or rhinorrhea.

Table 2: Probability of Clinically-Important Traumatic Brain Injuries Based on the Presence of Predictive Features for Children ≥2 Years[a]

Risk Category	Percentage of Children in this Category	Probability of ci-TBI
Altered Mental Status or Evidence of a Basilar Skull Fracture	14.0%	4.3%
Any of the Four Predictive Features Other than Altered Mental Status or Basilar Skull Fracture	27.7%	0.9%
None of the 6 Predictive Features	58.3%	<0.05%

[a]The numbers are similar for children <2 years except that the predictive features are different (see Table 1). For children <2 years, the highest risk category is "Altered Mental Status or Palpable Skull Fracture."

- in the validation sample, two children, both older than 2 years, who did not exhibit any of the 6 predictive features were ultimately found to have ciTBIs; both of these children were injured during sport-related activities, neither wore helmets, both had moderate headaches, and both had large frontal scalp hematomas; neither required neurosurgery

Criticisms and Limitations: Emergency departments were carefully selected for participation in this study. In real-world practice, clinicians – particularly those with less experience caring for children – may not be able to safely and effectively follow these prediction rules.

Because children change considerably between early infancy and two years of age, perhaps the prediction rule for this age group should be further stratified (e.g. a different rule for children <1 year and children ages 1 – 2 years).

Other Relevant Studies and Information:

- A follow-up analysis involving children in this study demonstrated that children who were observed in the emergency department for a period of time before a decision was made about obtaining a CT scan were less likely to receive a CT scan[230]

- Some studies have suggested that there may be as many as one case of lethal cancer due to radiation for every 1,000 to 5,000 head CT scans in children[231].

- Several other prediction rules for determining when CT scans are indicated in children with head trauma have also been developed[232].

SUMMARY AND IMPLICATIONS:

This study derived and validated prediction rules that can accurately identify children at very low risk for ci-TBI. The authors suggest that one way these rules could be applied is as follows:

- Children with none of the six predictive features are at very low risk (<0.05%) for ciTBI and typically do not require CT scans

---

230 Nigrovic et al. The effect of observation on cranial computed tomography utilization for children after blunt head trauma. Pediatrics. 2011 Jun;127(6):1067-73.

231 Brenner DJ and Hall EJ. Computed tomography – an increasing source of radiation exposure. N Engl J Med 2007;357:2277-84.

232 Maguire et al. Should a head-injured child receive a head CT scan? A systematic review of clinical prediction rules. Pediatrics. 2009;124(1):e145.

- Children with either of the two highest risk features – altered mental status or evidence of a skull fracture – are at high risk (approximately 4%) and should receive CT scans

- Children with any of the four predictive features other than altered mental status or evidence of a skull fracture have an intermediate risk for ci-TBI of approximately 0.9% and the decision about whether or not to obtain a CT should be individualized based on other factors such as the clinician's judgment, the number of predictive features present, serial evaluations of the patient over time, and the family's preferences

CLINICAL CASE: DETERMINING WHETHER OR NOT TO OBTAIN A HEAD CT

CASE HISTORY:

An 18 month old boy is brought to the emergency department by his parents after he fell off his parent's bed. The bed is approximately 3-4 feet off the ground, and he landed on the side of his head. The boy cried for several minutes after the fall, but he has been acting normally since. He did not lose consciousness after the fall.

On examination, he has a small abrasion over his right cheek, and he has tenderness to palpation over parts of the right parietal region of his scalp. He does not have any scalp hematomas, or palpable skull fractures. His neurologic examination is normal.

Based on the results of this study, should you order a CT scan to evaluate this boy for a traumatic brain injury?

SUGGESTED ANSWER:

The boy on this vignette has one of the six predictive features for a clinically important traumatic brain injury for children <2 years: he had a severe mechanism of injury (fall from a height >3 feet). Based on this study, his risk for a clinically important traumatic brain injury is approximately 0.9% (a more precise follow-up analysis estimates the risk for children <2 with a severe mechanism of injury but no other predictive features at 0.3%[233]). The authors of this study recommend that for children in this risk category, the decision about whether or not to obtain a head CT should be individualized based on the clinician's judgment and the family's preference.

As this boy's doctor, you might explain to his parents that the risk of brain injury is low. If you order a head CT scan, there is a small chance that you would detect an important abnormality, but most likely you would not. In addition, the radiation from the CT scan could be harmful. Thus, it would be reasonable either to proceed with the CT scan or to monitor the patient closely and only order a CT scan if the boy's condition worsens. You should engage the parents to determine which approach they are most comfortable with.

---

233 Nigrovic et al. Prevalence of Clinically Important Traumatic Brain Injuries in Children With Minor Blunt Head Trauma and Isolated Severe Injury Mechanisms. Arch Pediatr Adolesc Med. 2011 Dec 5.

SECTION 7:

NEUROLOGY AND PSYCHIATRY

THROMBOLYSIS 3 TO 4.5 HOURS AFTER AN ACUTE ISCHEMIC STROKE:

THE ECASS III TRIAL[234]

"… [A]lteplase given 3 to 4.5 hours after the onset of stroke symptoms was associated with a modest but significant improvement in the clinical outcome …"

- Hacke et al.[234]

Research Question: It has been established that thrombolysis with alteplase is effective when given within 3 hours of the onset of an acute ischemic stroke, however is alteplase effective when given 3 - 4.5 hours after the onset of a stroke?

---

234 Hacke et al. Thrombolysis with alteplase 3 to 4.5 hours after acute ischemic stroke. NEJM. 2008 Sep 25;359(13):1317-1329.

Funding: The Boehringer Ingelheim pharmaceutical company.

Year Study Began: 2003

Year Study Published: 2008

Study Location: More than 100 sites in Europe

Who Was Studied: Patients 18- 80 years old with an acute ischemic stroke presenting within 3 - 4.5 hours after the onset of symptoms.

Who Was Excluded: Patients with evidence of an intracranial hemorrhage on a CT or MRI scan of the head, those for whom the timing of symptom onset was unknown, those with major surgery or trauma within the previous 3 months, those with a systolic blood pressure >185 mm Hg or a diastolic pressure >110 mm Hg, and those on anticoagulants. In addition, patients with a "severe stroke", defined as a score >25 on the National Institutes of Health Stroke Scale[235] or "a stroke involving more than one third of the middle cerebral-artery territory" were excluded since strokes of this size are at high risk for hemorrhagic transformation.

How Many Patients: 821

Study Overview:

Figure 1: Summary of ECASS III's Design

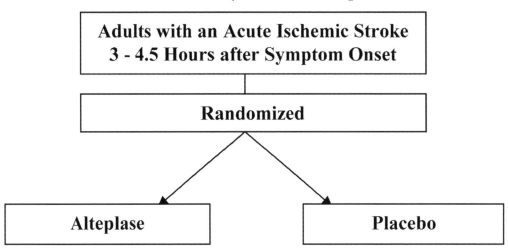

Study Intervention: Patients in the alteplase group received 0.9 mg per kg (max dose 90 mg) of alteplase intravenously. Patients in the placebo group

---

235 More information available at: http://www.strokecenter.org/trials/scales/nihss.html

received an intravenous placebo. Treatment with intravenous heparin, oral anticoagulants, and aspirin within 24 hours of administration of the study drug was prohibited, however prophylactic doses of heparin or low-molecular-weight heparin were permitted.

Follow-Up: 90 days

Endpoints: Primary outcome: disability as assessed using the modified Rankin scale[236]. Secondary outcomes: disability as assessed using a global disability scale consisting of scores on 4 individual disability scales (the modified Rankin scale, the Barthel Index, the National Institutes of Health Stroke Scale, and the Glasgow Outcome Scale); intracranial hemorrhage; and mortality.

Table 1: Modified Rankin Scale[237]

Score	Description
0	• No symptoms
1	• Able to carry out all usual activities
2	• "Unable to carry out all previous activities, but able to look after own affairs without assistance"
3	• "Requiring some help but able to walk without assistance"
4	• "Unable to walk without assistance and unable to attend to own bodily needs without assistance"
5	• "Bedridden, incontinent and requiring constant nursing care and attention"
6	• Dead

RESULTS:

- the median time for administration of the study medication following the onset of stroke symptoms was 3 hours and 59 minutes

236 Bonita et al. Modification of Rankin Scale: Recovery of motor function after stroke. Stroke 1988 Dec;19(12):1497-1500.

237 Further details at: http://www.strokecenter.org/trials/scales/rankin.html

Table 2: Summary of ECASS III's Key Findings

Outcome	Alteplase Group	Placebo Group	P Value
Favorable outcome on Rankin scale (score 0 or 1)	52.4%	45.2%	0.04
Mortality	7.7%	8.4%	0.68
Intracranial hemorrhage	27.0%	17.6%	0.001
Symptomatic intracranial hemorrhage	2.4%	0.2%	0.008

- the odds ratio for a positive outcome for alteplase on the global disability scale was 1.28 (95% CI, 1.00-1.65)

Criticisms and Limitations: Many emergency rooms including those involved in this trial have the capability of rapidly determining which patients are appropriate candidates for thrombolysis and administering the therapy quickly. In 'real world' settings, however, providing timely thrombolysis for patients presenting with acute strokes remains challenging.

Other Relevant Studies and Information:

- The NINDS trial established the benefit of alteplase for acute ischemic strokes within 3 hours of symptom onset[238]. Other trials have failed to show a benefit of thrombolysis up to 6 hours after symptom onset, however.

- Despite the fact that thrombolysis appears to be effective up to 4.5 hours after the onset of stroke symptoms, patients treated within the first 1.5 hours appear to have the best outcomes[239].

SUMMARY AND IMPLICATIONS:

The ECASS III trial established that thrombolysis with alteplase given up to 4.5 hours after the onset of stroke symptoms is modestly efficacious, however patients treated within the first 1.5 hours have the best outcomes.

---

238 The National Institute of Neurological Disorders and Stroke rt-PA Stroke Study Group. Tissue plasminogen activator for acute ischemic stroke. N Engl J Med. 1995;333(24):1581.

239 Hacke et al. Association of outcome with early stroke treatment: pooled analysis of ATLANTIS, ECAS, and NINDS rt-PA stroke trials. Lancet 2004;363:768-74.

CLINICAL CASE: THROMBOLYSIS FOR ACUTE ISCHEMIC STROKE

CASE HISTORY:

A 60 year old woman is rushed to the emergency room by ambulance after her daughter found her at home with slurred speech and weakness of her right arm. The woman called her daughter approximately 2.5 hours prior to arrival in the emergency room because she didn't feel right, but she cannot recall the exact time when her symptoms began: "Maybe an hour before I called my daughter? I really don't know."

On examination, the patient's vital signs are unremarkable. She has slurred speech and weakness of the right upper extremity.

An MRI of the brain, completed within 45 minutes of arrival in the emergency room, shows early ischemic changes involving approximately 20% of the territory of the right middle cerebral artery territory, but no hemorrhage.

Based on the results of ECASS III, should you treat this patient with thrombolytics?

SUGGESTED ANSWER:

The ECASS III trial established that thrombolysis with alteplase given up to 4.5 hours after the onset of stroke symptoms is modestly efficacious.

The patient in this vignette is likely experiencing an ischemic stroke and would be a good candidate for thrombolysis if her symptoms began within the previous 4.5 hours. The exact time when she developed symptoms is uncertain, but according to her best guess her symptoms began one hour prior to calling her daughter. An additional 2.5 hours elapsed before she arrived in the emergency room, followed by 45 minutes in the emergency room – for a total time of approximately 4 hours and 15 minutes. Thus, she should receive thrombolytics if the treatment can be administered immediately.

INITIAL TREATMENT OF DEPRESSION[240]

"[Patients] have an equal probability of recovering from [depression] whether treated pharmacologically or psychotherapeutically, even though the clinical progress will likely be slower with [psychotherapy]."

- Schulberg et al.[240]

Research Question: Is pharmacotherapy or psychotherapy more effective for the treatment of depression? Also, are these treatments superior to usual depression care from primary care doctors?

Funding: The National Institute of Mental Health.

Year Study Began: 1991

Year Study Published: 1996

Study Location: 4 outpatient clinics affiliated with the University of Pittsburgh

---

240 Schulberg et al. Treating major depression in primary care practice. Arch Gen Psychiatry. 1996;53:913-919.

Who Was Studied: Patients 18-64 who fulfilled DSM-III-R criteria[241] for current major depression and who had a minimum score of 13 on the 17-item Hamilton Rating Scale-Depression (HRS-D)[242]. These determinations were made by a psychiatrist.

The HRS-D scale is described below. The DSM-III-R criteria for depression, which are similar to the DSM-IV criteria, include the presence of dysphoria along with most of the following other symptoms:

- loss of interest

- appetite disturbance

- sleep disturbance

- psychomotor change

- loss of energy

- feelings of guilt

- thinking or concentration disturbance

- thoughts of death or suicide

Who Was Excluded: Patients with another medical or psychiatric condition preventing random assignment to one of the treatment groups. In addition, patients receiving current treatment for a mood disorder were ineligible.

How Many Patients: 276

Study Overview:

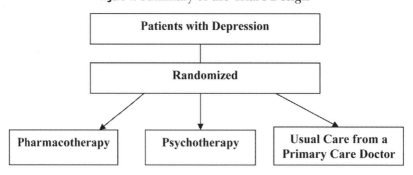

Figure 1: Summary of the Trial's Design

---

241 American Psychiatric Association. Diagnostic and Statistical Manual of Mental Disorders, Third Edition, Revised. Washington, DC: Amnerican Psychiatric Association;1987.

242 Hamilton M. A rating scale for depression. J Neurol Neurosurg Psychiatry 1960; 23:56–62

Study Intervention: Patients assigned to receive pharmacotherapy were treated with nortriptyline by family practitioners or general internists trained in pharmacotherapy. Each patient was treated within his or her regular medical clinic, however the prescribing doctor was not the patient's usual doctor. Patients were initially started on a nortriptyline dose of 25 mg, and were seen weekly or every two weeks for medication titration. Once patients showed clinical improvement and had therapeutic nortriptyline serum levels (190-570 nmol/L), they were transitioned to monthly visits for an additional 6 months.

Patients assigned to psychotherapy were treated with interpersonal psychotherapy by psychiatrists and psychologists. Patients received 16 weekly sessions at their regular medical clinic followed by 4 monthly maintenance sessions.

Patients assigned to usual care were treated by their primary care physicians according to each physician's regular practices.

Follow-Up: 8 months

Endpoints: Mean scores on the HRS-D. In addition, the authors determined the proportion of patients in each group who had "recovered" from depression as indicated by an HRS-D score ≤7.

The HRS-D is a commonly used depression scoring system based on the severity of depression symptoms. It is administered by clinicians. A score ≥20 is commonly considered to indicate depression of moderate severity. Study patients were required to have a minimum HSR-D score of 13, and the mean baseline score of study patients was 23. Below is a sample item on the 17-item survey:

> ➤ Depressed Mood:
>
> > 0- absent
> >
> > 1- these feeling states indicated only on questioning
> >
> > 2- these feelings states spontaneously reported verbally
> >
> > 3- communicates feeling states non-verbally, i.e. through facial expressions, posture, voice and tendency to weep
> >
> > 4- patient reports virtually only these feeling states in his/her spontaneous verbal and non-verbal communication

RESULTS:

- the mean age of study patients was 38, and over 80% were female

- the mean baseline HRS-D score for study patients was 23

- 33% of patients assigned to pharmacotherapy completed all 8 months of therapy vs. 42% of patients assigned to psychotherapy

- in the usual care group, 63% of patients received some form of mental health treatment and 45% received an antidepressant within 2 months of the trial's onset

Table 1: Summary of the Trial's Key Findings

Outcome	Nortriptyline Group	Psychotherapy Group	Usual Care Group	Significance Testing[a]
Mean HRS-D Score At Trial Completion	9.0	9.3	13.1	Nortriptyline and psychotherapy were superior to usual care; there was no difference between nortriptyline and psychotherapy
Depression Recovery Rate (HRS-D ≤7)	48%	46%	18%	Nortriptyline and psychotherapy were superior to usual care; there was no difference between nortriptyline and psychotherapy

[a]Actual p values not reported.

- although there were no significant differences in depression symptoms between patients assigned to nortriptyline vs. psychotherapy at the completion of the trial (8 months of follow-up), improvement was more rapid among patients who received nortriptyline

Criticisms and Limitations: Primary care doctors treating patients assigned to the usual care group were not always informed immediately that their patients had been diagnosed with depression. This may have caused a delay in treatment initiation, potentially leading to poorer outcomes among patients in the usual care group.

Depression therapies have evolved since this trial was conducted. For example, selective serotonin reuptake inhibitors (SSRIs) – not nortriptyline – are now first line pharmacotherapy for depression due to their more favorable side-effect profile[243]. More recent trials comparing SSRIs with psychotherapy have come to similar conclusions as this one, however[244,245].

Finally, just 33% of patients assigned to pharmacotherapy and 42% of patients assigned to psychotherapy completed all 8 months of therapy. This demonstrates the challenges of treating patients with depression with either of these modalities.

Other Relevant Studies and Information:

- Other trials comparing antidepressant medications with psychotherapy have come to similar conclusions as this one[244,245,246].

- Some studies have suggested that a combination of pharmacotherapy and psychotherapy may be slightly more beneficial than either treatment alone, particularly for patients with severe chronic depression[247].

- Guidelines from the Agency for Health Care Policy and Research conclude that either medications or psychotherapy are appropriate initial therapy for mild or moderate depression, however severely depressed patients should receive medications[248].

SUMMARY AND IMPLICATIONS:

243 Mulrow et al. Efficacy of newer medications for treating depression in primary care patients. Am J Med. 2000;108(1):54.

244 Chilvers et al. Antidepressant drugs and generic counseling for treatment of major depression in primary care: randomized trial with patient preference arms. The British Medical Journal. 2001;322:1-5.

245 DeRubeis et al. Cognitive therapy vs. medications in the treatment of moderate to severe depression. Arch Gen Psychiatry. 2005;62:409-416.

246 Schulberg et al. The effectiveness of psychotherapy in treating depressive disorders in primary care practice: clinical and cost perspectives. Gen Hosp Psychiatry. 2002;24(4):203.

247 Pampallona et al. Combined pharmacotherapy and psychological treatment for depression: a systematic review. Arch Gen Psychiatry. 2004;61(7):714.

248 Depression Guideline Panel. Depression in Primary Care: Treatment of Major Depression: Clinical Practice Guideline. US Dept of Health and Human Services, Public Health Service, Agency for Health Care Policy and Research. AHCPR publication 93-0551, Rockville, MD 1993.

In primary care patients with depression, initial treatment with psychotherapy and pharmacotherapy (nortriptyline) were equally efficacious, however clinical improvement was slightly faster with pharmacotherapy. The psychotherapy and pharmacotherapy protocols used in this trial were both superior to usual care from primary care doctors, highlighting the need for standardized depression treatment.

CLINICAL CASE: INITIAL TREATMENT OF DEPRESSION

CASE HISTORY:

A 52 year old woman visits your primary care office because she has been feeling "down" for the past two months. She says that life's stresses have been wearing on her. She has had several previous depressive episodes, but has never sought medical attention before. She reports that she has not been sleeping well, her energy level has been low, and that she frequently feels guilty and inadequate. She denies problems with her appetite, psychomotor changes, difficulty concentrating, suicidal ideations, or frequent thoughts of death.

Based on the results of this trial, what treatment options would you consider for this patient?

SUGGESTED ANSWER:

This trial demonstrated that psychotherapy and pharmacotherapy were equally efficacious for the initial management of depression, however clinical improvement was slightly faster with pharmacotherapy.

The patient in this vignette has symptoms consistent with mild depression. She could be treated with either psychotherapy – assuming high quality psychotherapy services are available – or pharmacotherapy (likely a selective serotonin reuptake inhibitor because of the favorable side-effects profile). After explaining the options to the patient, you should ask which approach she prefers.

BEHAVIORAL VS. PHARMACOLOGICAL TREATMENT FOR INSOMNIA IN THE ELDERLY[249]

"[These] findings indicate that behavioral and pharmacological therapies, alone or in combination, are effective in short-term management of late-life insomnia ... Follow-up results showed that behavior therapy yielded the most durable improvements ..."

- Morin et al.[249]

Research Question: Which is better for treating insomnia in the elderly: cognitive-behavioral therapy (CBT), medications, or a combination of the two?

Funding: The National Institute of Mental Health.

---

249 Morin et al. Behavioral and pharmacological therapies for late-life insomnia: A randomized controlled trial. JAMA. 1999;281(11):991-999.

Year Study Began: mid 1990's

Year Study Published: 1999

Study Location: An academic medical center in Virginia

Who Was Studied: Adults ≥55 with either sleep-onset insomnia or sleep-maintenance insomnia for at least six months. Sleep onset insomnia was defined as latency of sleep onset for more than 30 minutes at least three nights a week, while sleep-maintenance insomnia was defined as waking after falling asleep for more than 30 minutes at least three nights a week. To be eligible, patients also were required to have daytime symptoms such as fatigue.

Study patients were recruited through letters to physicians and newspaper advertisements. Volunteers underwent an intensive screening evaluation by a sleep specialist, a psychologist, and a physician to determine which ones were eligible. Fewer than half of the volunteers ultimately were found to be eligible.

Who Was Excluded: Patients whose insomnia was due to a medical condition or a medication, those with sleep apnea, those regularly taking sleep medications, those with a severe mental health disturbance, those living in a nursing home or other facility, and those with cognitive impairment.

How Many Patients: 78

Study Overview:

Figure 1: Summary of the Trial's Design

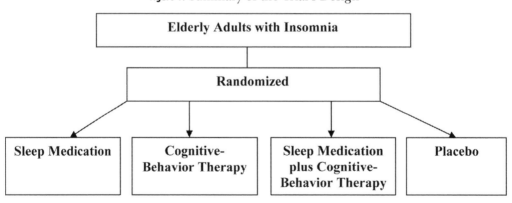

Study Intervention: Patients assigned to receive CBT were offered weekly 90-minute group therapy sessions led by a clinical psychologist for eight weeks. During these sessions, patients were taught to restrict time in bed in order to increase the proportion of time spent sleeping. In addition, patients were taught to use the bedroom only for sleep and to leave the bedroom whenever they could not fall asleep within 15-20 minutes. Finally, the CBT sessions addressed faulty beliefs about sleep (for example that everyone must sleep 8 hours every night) and provided education about sleep hygiene and how sleep patterns change with normal aging.

Patients assigned to the medication group were prescribed temazepam to be taken 1 hour before bedtime. Patients met weekly with a psychiatrist to discuss medication management. The initial temazepam dose was 7.5 mg, and this could gradually be increased by the physician if necessary to a maximum of 30 mg. Patients were encouraged to use temazepam at least 2-3 nights per week and were given enough medication to use every night if they chose to.

Patients assigned to the combined CBT plus medication group received both of the above treatments.

Patients assigned to the placebo group received placebo pills according to the same schedule as patients in the temazepam group.

At the conclusion of the therapy, patients resumed regular treatment by their physician, however follow-up monitoring continued for a total of 24 months.

Follow-Up: 24 months

Endpoints: 1) Sleep time as measured by sleep diaries kept by patients and by polysomnography; and 2) Scores on the Sleep Impairment Index, a survey that assesses the clinical severity of insomnia with respect to sleep disturbance, daytime functioning, distress caused by the sleep problem, and overall satisfaction with sleep.

RESULTS:

- 63% of patients had mixed insomnia (i.e. both sleep-onset and sleep-maintenance insomnia), while 28% had only sleep-maintenance insomnia, and 6% had only sleep-onset insomnia

- The average duration of insomnia symptoms among study patients was 17 years, and 77% of patients had previously used sleep medications

- Treatment compliance in all groups was high: patients assigned to receive CBT attended 97% of the sessions, and patients assigned to receive medication took the medication approximately 75% of all nights

Summary of the Trial's Key Findings:

- Sleep patterns as measured with sleep diaries improved with all three active treatments compared to placebo (P<0.05)

- Sleep patterns as measured with polysomnography followed a similar pattern, however only combined therapy resulted in statistically significant improvements compared to placebo (CBT and medications resulted in non-significant improvements)

- The combined treatment appeared more effective than either CBT or medication alone, however the difference did not reach statistical significance

- CBT and combined treatment led to greater improvements on the patient-reported Sleep Impairment Index than did medication (P=0.01) or placebo (P=0.002)

- Improvements in sleep patterns were better sustained after 24 months with CBT than with pharmacotherapy

Table 1: Total Sleep Time in Minutes[a]

	Cognitive-Behavior Therapy Group	Medication Group	Combined Therapy Group	Placebo Group
Pretreatment	322	340	290	331
Posttreatment	352	384	332	351
24-month Follow-up	387	352	331	331

[a]These data are from sleep diaries kept by patients. Polysomnography data followed a similar pattern.

Criticisms and Limitations: This study involved a carefully selected group of patients who were extremely compliant with the study protocol. These findings may not apply to patients outside of a research setting. For example, many "real-world" patients might not attend CBT sessions as reliably as these patients did.

In this study, CBT involved eight group sessions with a clinical psychologist. Such therapy may not be available in all settings, and it is also expensive.

For obvious reasons, neither the patients who received CBT nor their treating clinicians were blinded to the treatment assignment. It is possible that the lack of blinding could have biased the results. For example, patients in the CBT group may have been more likely to report improvements in their sleep patterns simply because they knew they were receiving a "real" treatment rather than placebo.

Because the sample size for this study was small (78 patients), the study was underpowered to detect small difference in the effectiveness of the three treatment options.

Other Relevant Studies and Information:

- Trials comparing CBT with medication for insomnia in both young adults and the elderly have generally come to similar conclusions as this trial[250,251,252]

- In a trial comparing CBT vs. CBT combined with medication (zolpidem), the combined treatment led to a slightly better initial response than CBT alone, however patients in the combined group who were ultimately tapered off medication had the best response[253]

- Most experts recommend CBT, either alone or (in severe cases) in combination with medication as first-line treatment for chronic insomnia; when medication is used, it should ideally only be given for several weeks

SUMMARY AND IMPLICATIONS:

All three treatments – CBT, medication, and combination therapy – improved symptoms of insomnia more than placebo. Combination therapy initially appeared to be most effective, however both combination therapy and CBT alone led to greater improvements in patient-reported symptoms than medication alone. Importantly, CBT appeared to produce the best outcomes with long term follow-up.

---

250 Jacobs et al. Cognitive behavior therapy and pharmacotherapy for insomnia: a randomized controlled trial and direct comparison. *Arch Intern Med.* 2004;164(17):1888-1896.

251 Sivertsen et al. Cognitive behavioral therapy vs. zopiclone for treatment of chronic primary insomnia in older adults. JAMA 2006;295(24):2851-2858.

252 McClusky et al. Efficacy of behavioral vs. triazolam treatment in persistent sleep-onset insomnia. *Am J Psychiatry.* 1991;148(1):121-126.

253 Morin et al. Cognitive behavioral therapy, singly and combined with medication, for persistent insomnia: a randomized controlled trial. JAMA. 2009;301(19):2005.

CLINICAL CASE: INSOMNIA IN THE ELDERLY

CASE HISTORY:

A 76 year old woman presents to your office two weeks after her husband unexpectedly passed away to ask if you can do anything to help with her insomnia. Upon further questioning, you discover that she has had trouble sleeping for several years, however the problem has become acutely worse since her husband died. She reports that she "hasn't slept a wink" in over a week, and constantly feels tired and irritable during the day. In addition, the woman appears sad.

Based on the results of this trial, how should you treat her insomnia?

SUGGESTED ANSWER:

This patient has chronic insomnia that has become acutely worse since her husband passed away. Because the acute symptoms are extremely bothersome, it would be appropriate to prescribe her a sleep medication such as a benzodiazepine or zolpidem. The medication should be used cautiously because elderly patients are prone to side effects such as over-sedation. In addition, it would be important to monitor the patient's psychological state closely. While it is appropriate for her to feel sad, elderly patients are prone to depression. You might suggest that she come for regular clinic visits or telephone consultations during this difficult time. In addition, you might encourage her to spend time with family and friends if possible.

In addition to treating the acute insomnia, the patient should receive CBT for the chronic insomnia. Specifically, she might try using the bedroom only to sleep, leaving the bedroom when she has difficulty falling asleep, improving her sleep hygiene, and time restriction in bed. Such treatment – which could be delayed until the patient's grief begins to subside – will ultimately have a more lasting impact on her sleep patterns than medication.

SECTION 8:

SYSTEMS BASED PRACTICE

THE GROUP HEALTH MEDICAL HOME DEMONSTRATION[254]

"Group Health's experience ... suggests that primary care enhancements, in the form of the medical home, hold promise for controlling costs, improving quality, and better meeting the needs of patients and care teams."

- Reid et al.[254]

Research Question: Can a primary care practice improve healthcare quality and/ or lower costs by reorganizing according to the principles of the medical home model, which emphasize continuity of care with a personal physician, team-based and integrated care, and enhanced access to care?

Funding: The Group Health Cooperative and the Group Health Permanente medical group

Year Study Began: 2006

---

254 Reid et al. The Group Health medical home at year two: cost savings, higher patient satisfaction, and less burnout for providers. Health Aff (Millwood). 2010 May;29(5):835-43.

Year Study Published: 2010

Study Location: A clinic at the Group Health Cooperative in the Seattle, Washington area

Who Was Studied: The patients and providers at a primary care internal medicine practice in Seattle that piloted a practice transformation in accordance with the medical home model. The clinic is owned and operated by the Group Health Cooperative, a non-profit healthcare system. The clinic has approximately 9,200 adult patients. Other Group Health clinics served as controls.

How Many Patients: Approximately 7,000 adult patients who were continuously enrolled at the medical home clinic during the study period. The control group consisted of approximately 200,000 patients continuously enrolled in 19 nearby Group Health clinics.

Study Overview: Patient and provider satisfaction were compared between the medical home clinic and two control clinics that were "selected based on similarities in size, Medicare enrollment, and leadership stability." In addition, healthcare quality, utilization, and costs were compared between the medical home clinic and the 19 control clinics.

Study Intervention: The principles for the medical home redesign were developed using ideas from national experts as well as from two workshops involving Group Health physicians, staff, patients, and researchers. As part of the redesign, clinical staff were organized into care teams consisting of physician leaders, medical assistants, licensed practical nurses, physician assistants or nurse practitioners, registered nurses, and a clinical pharmacist. The care teams held daily "huddles" to promote care planning and coordination, and to troubleshoot problems.

Table 1: Summary of the Group Health Clinic Transformation

General Changes
- Physician panel sizes were reduced from 2,300 to a target of 1,800
- Patient visit times were increased from 20 to 30 minutes
- Physicians were exempted from productivity-based incentives

Information Technology Changes
- E-mail and telephone communication between patients and providers was encouraged
- Patients were encouraged to check their lab results and request medication refills online
- Patients were enabled and encouraged to view "after visit summaries" from the electronic health record

Chronic Care Management
- Clinicians consistently used electronic registries, health maintenance reminders, and best-practice alerts
- Care plans were developed for patients with chronic diseases
- Self-care for patients with chronic conditions was promoted through group visits, behavior-change programs, and peer-led chronic illness workshops

Visit Preparation
- Patients were contacted prior to their visits to discuss concerns
- Clinicians regularly reviewed patient charts to monitor lab test results, referral notes, and unmet care needs

Patient Outreach
- Patients received follow-up after all hospitalizations and emergency and urgent care visits
- Patients were contacted when unmet care needs were identified
- Patients were contacted for medication monitoring and abnormal test results

Practice Management Changes
- Patient phone calls were forwarded directly to the care team
- Team performance was continuously tracked, and problems were addressed in a systematic fashion during team huddles

Follow-Up: Two years

Endpoints: Patient satisfaction as assessed by patient surveys; provider burnout as assessed by surveys of physicians and other clinical staff; quality of care scores based on 22 measures from the Healthcare Effectiveness Information Set (HEDIS); and healthcare utilization and costs.

RESULTS:

Patient Experience:

- during the study period, patients in the medical home clinic reported modestly better care experiences than those in the control clinics

- as an example, survey scores for care coordination (on a scale with 100 possible points) increased from 80.7 to 83.9 in the medical home clinic vs. 77.4 to 78.9 in the control clinics

Provider Burnout:

- at baseline, scores on the provider survey were similar among staff at the medical home and control clinics

- at the end of the two year study period, emotional exhaustion scores and depersonalization scores, but not personal accomplishment scores, were significantly better among staff at the medical home clinic

Quality of Care:

- the average patient in the medical home clinic achieved 68.7% of the HEDIS measures at the start of the study and 75.9% at the end

- the average patient in the control clinics achieved 64.3% of the HEDIS measures at the start of the study and 70.3% at the end

- the improvement in the medical home clinic was 1.3 percentage points better than in the control clinics (P<0.05)

Healthcare Utilization and Costs:

- patients in the medical home clinic had 6% fewer primary care visits, but more email and phone communication than patients in the control clinics

- patients in the medical home clinic made 29% fewer visits for emergency and urgent care appointments than patients in the control clinics

- all-cause hospitalizations were 6% lower in the medical home clinic

- estimated total costs were $10.30 lower per patient per month at the medical home clinic, though this difference did not reach statistical significance (P=0.08)

- the authors estimate that for every dollar spent on recruiting and hiring additional staff to implement the medical home, Group Health received $1.50 in return (this estimate does not include investments in other system-wide improvements or information technology that had previously been implemented)

Criticisms and Limitations: Since this was not a randomized trial, confounding factors may have influenced the results. For example, although the researchers attempted to control for difference between the medical home and control clinics, it is possible that the lower utilization rates and cost at the medical home clinic resulted not from the changes that were implemented but rather from other factors such as a healthier population or more enthusiastic staff at the medical home clinic. In addition, the surveys were only completed by a fraction of patients and clinic staff, and therefore only reflect the opinions of those who were willing to complete the surveys.

SUMMARY AND IMPLICATIONS:

Despite the limitations described above, the Group Health medical home demonstration suggests that investment in primary care has the potential to improve healthcare quality and perhaps lower costs. In addition, the changes Group Health implemented appeared to have favorable effects on patient and, especially, staff satisfaction.

CLINICAL CASE: THE GROUP HEALTH MEDICAL HOME DEMONSTRATION

CASE HISTORY:

In response to national health care reform, a primary care internal medicine clinic plans to transform itself into a medical home. The clinic provides its patients with email addresses for all the doctors, and promises patients that they will receive responses to their emailed questions within 24 hours. In addition, all patients are promised that they will be able to receive same-day appointments whenever they want. In order to support these extra services, the clinic plans to incentivize doctors to be more efficient by basing their salaries largely on productivity.

After reading about the Group Health Medical Home Demonstration, what do you think the impact of this program will be?

SUGGESTED ANSWER:

The Group Health Medical Home Demonstration led to a reduction in ER and hospitalization rates, as well as improvements in patient and staff satisfaction. However, Group Health provided considerable resources to support its medical home transformation (e.g. the hiring of additional physicians and other staff members). Other attempts at implementing medical homes that have not provided adequate resources have not resulted in similar favorable effects. Therefore, the program described in this vignette is unlikely to be successful.

A PROGRAM TO IMPROVE CARE COORDINATION AT HOSPITAL DISCHARGE:

PROJECT RED[255]

"The [Project] RED intervention decreased hospital utilization (combined emergency department visits and readmissions) within 30 days of discharge by about 30% among patients on a general medicine service of an urban, academic medical center."

- Jack et al.[255]

Research Question: Is it possible to reduce the rate of repeat emergency room and hospital visits after discharge by improving care coordination?

---

255 Jack et al. A reengineered hospital discharge program to decrease rehospitalization. Annals of Internal Medicine. 2009;150:178-187.

Funding: The Agency for Healthcare Research and Quality and the National Heart, Lung, and Blood Institute, National Institutes of Health.

Year Study Began: 2004

Year Study Published: 2009

Study Location: Boston Medical Center, Boston, Massachusetts

Who Was Studied: Adults admitted to the general medicine service of an urban, academic medical center that serves an "ethnically diverse patient population."

Who Was Excluded: Patients without a home telephone, those unable to "comprehend study details and the consent process in English," those on a suicide watch, and those who were blind or deaf. In addition, patients were excluded if they were not discharged home (e.g. if they were discharged to a nursing facility).

How Many Patients: 749

Study Overview:

Figure 1: Summary of the Trial's Design

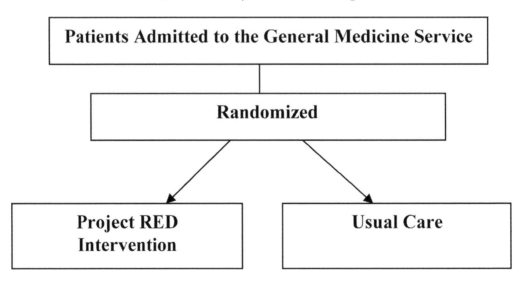

Study Intervention: Patients in the Project RED (Reengineered Discharge) group were assigned to nurse discharge advocates who provided the patients with the following services and assistance during the hospitalization:

- Education about their condition

- Assistance with post-discharge appointment scheduling and planning

- Education about medications and medication reconciliation upon discharge

- Education about how to address post-discharge problems (e.g. whom to contact)

At the time of discharge, the advocates gave each patient a written discharge plan listing the reason for hospitalization, the discharge medication list, contact information for the patient's ambulatory care providers, and information about post-discharge appointments and testing. The discharge advocates transmitted the post-discharge care plan and the hospital discharge summary to each patient's ambulatory providers.

Two to four days after discharge, a clinical pharmacist called each patient "to reinforce the discharge plan, review medications, and solve problems."

Patients in the control group received usual hospital and post-discharge care.

Follow-Up: 30 days

Endpoints: Primary outcome: emergency room and hospital visits within 30 days of hospital discharge. Secondary outcomes: patients' knowledge about their discharge diagnoses; the percentage of patients visiting their primary care doctors after discharge; and "self-reported preparedness for discharge."

RESULTS:

- among patients in the Project RED group, 83% were discharged with a written discharge plan and 91% had their discharge information transmitted to their primary care doctors within 24 hours of discharge

- after discharge, pharmacists were able to reach 62% of patients in the Project RED group by telephone, and over half of the patients who were contacted had medication problems requiring "corrective action"

- Project RED discharge advocates spent an estimated 87.5 minutes per patient, while pharmacists spent an estimated 26 minutes per patient

Table 1: Summary of the Trial's Key Findings

Outcome	Control Group	Project RED Group	P Value
Total Hospital and Emergency Room Visits After Discharge	0.451[a]	0.314[a]	0.009
Emergency Room Visits	0.245[a]	0.165[a]	0.014
Hospital Visits	0.207[a]	0.149[a]	0.090
Patients Able to Identify Their Discharge Diagnoses	70%	79%	0.017
Patients Visiting Their Primary Doctors after Discharge	44%	62%	<0.001
Patients Reporting that they Felt Prepared for Discharge	55%	65%	0.013

[a]Mean number of visits per patient per month.

- Project RED was most effective in preventing emergency room and hospital visits among patients with the highest hospital utilization during the previous six months

- overall, Project RED lowered health care costs by an average of $412 per patient (mainly by preventing emergency room and hospital visits); the authors did not indicate whether these savings offset the program costs, however

Criticisms and Limitations: Because of staffing limitations, the nurse discharge advocates were only able to enroll 2-3 patients per day, and didn't enroll any patients on some weekends and holidays.

Since Project RED involved multiple components (i.e. education in the hospital, post-discharge planning, and post-discharge outreach), it is not clear which component of the program was responsible for its success.

The Project RED intervention might not have been as effective in other healthcare settings. For example, patients of higher socioeconomic status might not require as much assistance with post-discharge planning.

Other Relevant Studies and Information:

- Other studies have also demonstrated that care coordination programs at the time of hospital discharge can reduce the rate of repeat emergency room and hospital visits[256,257]; not all such programs have been successful, however[258,259]

SUMMARY AND IMPLICATIONS:

The Project RED program substantially reduced repeat emergency room and hospital visits by improving care coordination at the time of hospital discharge.

CLINICAL CASE: CARE COORDINATION AT HOSPITAL DISCHARGE

CASE HISTORY:

A community hospital wants to improve care coordination for its patients at the time of discharge. What are the challenges to implementing a program like Project RED?

SUGGESTED ANSWER:

Perhaps the largest obstacle to implementing a program like Project RED is financial since it is not clear where the funding for such a program should come from. Improving care coordination does not generate revenue for the hospital (in fact, it could have the opposite effect by reducing emergency

---

256 Coleman et al. The care transitions intervention: results of a random controlled trial. Arch Intern Med. 2006;166:1822-8.

257 Naylor et al. Comprehensive discharge planning and home follow-up of hospitalized elders: a randomized clinical trial. JAMA. 1999;281:613-20.

258 Weinberger et al. Does increased access to primary care reduce hospital readmissions? Veterans Affairs Cooperative Study Group on Primary Care and Hospital Readmission. NEJM. 1996;334:1441-7.

259 Shepperd et al. Discharge planning from hospital to home. Cochrane Database Syst Rev. 2004:CD000313.

room and hospital visits). Moreover, insurance companies do not typically reimburse for programs like Project RED.

The Medicare program is currently trying to restructure financial incentives to promote programs like Project RED that improve health care quality and efficiency. For example, Medicare is beginning to penalize hospitals with high readmission rates in an attempt to promote care coordination at discharge.

REDUCING CATHETER-RELATED BLOOD STREAM INFECTIONS IN THE INTENSIVE CARE UNIT:

THE KEYSTONE ICU PROJECT[260]

"As part of the Michigan statewide patient-safety initiative, we implemented a simple and inexpensive intervention to reduce [catheter-related bloodstream infections] in 103 ICUs. Coincident with the intervention, the median rate of infection decreased from 2.7 per 1000 catheter-days at baseline to 0 within the first 3 months after the implementation of the intervention."

- Pronovost et al.[260]

---

260 Pronovost et al. An intervention to decrease catheter-related bloodstream infections in the ICU. N Engl J Med. 2006 Dec 28;355(26):2725-32.

Research Question: Can rates of catheter-related blood stream infections be reduced by implementing a safety initiative involving 5 simple infection-control measures by intensive care unit (ICU) staff?

Sponsor: The U.S. Agency for Healthcare Research and Quality

Year Study Began: 2003

Year Study Published: 2006

Study Location: 103 intensive care units in 67 Michigan hospitals

Who Was Studied: Patients from 103 intensive care units in 67 Michigan hospitals, representing 85% of all ICU beds in Michigan. ICUs included medical, surgical, cardiac, neurologic, surgical trauma units, and one pediatric unit.

Who Was Excluded: Data from 4 ICUs were excluded because these hospitals did not track the necessary data, and data from 1 ICU were merged and included with data from another ICU. In addition, 34 hospitals in Michigan chose not to participate in the project.

How Many Patients: A total of 375,757 catheter-days, which refers to the total number of days in which catheters were in place for all study patients. For example, a patient with a catheter in place for 7 days would represent 7 catheter days.

Study Overview: As part of the Michigan Keystone ICU project, participating ICUs implemented a series of patient-safety interventions including the use of a daily goals sheet to improve staff communication, a program to improve the culture of safety among staff, and an intervention to reduce the rate of catheter-related blood stream infections. This analysis focuses on the intervention aimed at preventing catheter-related blood stream infections.

Rates of blood stream infections in participating ICUs were monitored for a 3 month period prior to implementation of the safety initiative and for an 18-month period afterwards.

Study Intervention: In preparation for implementation of the safety initiative, each ICU designated at least one physician and one nurse as team leaders. Team leaders received training in the "science of safety" and on the components of the initiative through "conference calls every other week, coaching by research staff, and statewide meetings twice a year." The team leaders, along with each hospital's infection-control staff, led implementation of the safety initiative at their respective institutions.

The safety initiative involved the promotion of 5 simple measures for preventing blood stream infections:

- Hand washing

- Using sterile drapes during the insertion of central venous catheters

- Cleaning the skin with chlorhexidine disinfectant prior to catheter insertion

- Avoiding the femoral site for central line insertion whenever possible

- Removing unnecessary catheters

These practices were encouraged in the following ways:

- Clinicians received education about the harms of blood-stream infections and the importance of following infection control measures

- A cart was created in each ICU with the necessary supplies for central line insertion

- The central line carts included a checklist reminding staff to follow the preventive measures, and clinicians were instructed to complete the checklists whenever they placed central lines

- During daily ICU rounds, teams discussed the removal of unnecessary catheters

- Clinician teams received regular feedback on the rates of blood stream infections among their patients

- ICU staff were empowered to stop central line insertion if they observed that the preventive measures were not being followed (i.e. nurses and other staff had the authority to stop doctors who were not following the safety measures)

Follow-Up: 18 months

Endpoints: Change in the rate of catheter-related blood stream infections before and after the initiative began.

RESULTS:

- The percentage of hospital ICUs stocking chlorhexidine in central line kits increased from 19% prior to the start of the initiative to 64% 6 weeks afterwards

Table 1: Key Findings from the Keystone ICU Project

Time	Median Infections Per 1000 Catheter Days at Study Hospitals[a]	Range of Infection Rates Per 1000 Catheter Days at Study Hospitals[b]	P Value for Comparison with Baseline Rates
Baseline	2.7	0.6 - 4.8	–
During Implementation	1.6	0.0 - 4.4	≤0.05
After Implementation			
0-3 months	0	0.0 - 3.0	≤0.002
16-18 months	0	0.0 - 2.4	≤0.002

[a]Catheter-days refer to the total number of days in which catheters were in place for all study patients. For example, a patient with a catheter in place for 7 days would represent 7 catheter days.
[b]The highest and lowest infection rates among study hospitals.

- Mean infection rates decreased continuously throughout the study period, i.e. the safety initiative became increasingly more effective throughout the study period

- The safety initiative was effective among both teaching and non-teaching hospitals, as well as among both large (≥200 beds) and small (<200 beds) hospitals, though it appeared to be slightly more effective at small hospitals

Criticisms and Limitations: Because there were no control ICUs that did not implement the safety initiative, it is not possible to prove that the initiative – rather than other factors – was responsible for the observed reduction in infections. The fact that infection rates didn't decrease substantially in other states during the same time period argues against an alternative explanation, however.

It is possible that the number of reported infections during the study period decreased simply because hospital staff changed the way that they diagnosed catheter-related blood stream infections. For example, hospital staff may have under-reported these infections during the study period simply because they knew that infection rates were being closely tracked. The authors believe this is unlikely, however, because "infection rates were collected and reported" according to pre-specified criteria by "hospital infection-control practitioners who were independent of the ICU staff."

It is not known how well ICU staff followed each component of the initiative, nor is it known which component was most important for reducing infection rates. For example, it is possible that most of the observed benefit resulted from a single component of the initiative such as the use of chlorhexidine disinfectant.

Finally, it is not known how much time, effort, and cost each ICU had to invest to comply with the intervention. Resource utilization was likely modest, however, because the intervention was simple and did not require expensive equipment or supplies.

ADDITIONAL INFORMATION:

- A follow up analysis showed that the reduction in catheter-related bloodstream infections in Michigan was sustained for an additional 18 months (total follow up of 36 months)[261]

- A follow up analysis also showed that implementation of the safety initiative was associated with a reduction in all-cause ICU mortality among Medicare patients in Michigan compared with the surrounding states[262]

- A cost analysis examining data from 6 hospitals that were part of the Keystone ICU project suggested that the intervention saved money for the health care system: the average cost of the intervention was $3,375 per infection averted, however catheter-related blood steam infections typically cost approximately $12,000 - $54,000 to treat[263]

- The model used in the Keystone ICU initiative has been successfully implemented in other states including Rhode Island[264] and Hawaii[265]

261 Pronovost et al. Sustaining reductions in catheter related bloodstream infections in Michigan intensive care units: observational study. BMJ. 2010;340:c309.

262 Lipitz-Snyderman et al. Impact of a statewide intensive care unit quality improvement initiative on hospital mortality and length of stay: retrospective comparative analysis. BMJ. 2011 Jan 28;342.

263 Waters et al. The business case for quality: economic analysis of the Michigan Keystone Patient Safety Program in ICUs. Am J Med Qual. 2011 Sep-Oct;26(5):333-9.

264 DePalo et al. The Rhode Island ICU collaborative: a model for reducing central line-associated bloodstream infection and ventilator-associated pneumonia statewide. Qual Saf Health Care. 2010 Dec;19(6):555-61.

265 Lin et al. Eradicating Central Line-Associated Bloodstream Infections Statewide: The Hawaii Experience. Am J Med Qual. 2011 Sep 14.

- Simple checklist protocols to reduce complication rates among surgical patients have also proven to be highly effective[266,267]

- Studies have suggested that the rates of other hospital-acquired infections such ventilator-associated pneumonia can be greatly reduced with the use of simple checklist protocols[268,269]

- Despite the successes of these safety initiatives, many hospitals in the U.S. and around the world do not consistently utilize these simple measures

SUMMARY AND IMPLICATIONS:

Implementation of a safety initiative involving 5 simple infection-control measures by ICU staff was associated with a substantial reduction in catheter-related blood stream infections. While it is not certain that the safety initiative – rather than other factors – was responsible for the observed reduction, the study provides strong evidence that this safety initiative should be implemented widely.

REDUCING CATHETER-RELATED BLOOD STREAM INFECTIONS IN THE INTENSIVE CARE UNIT

CASE HISTORY:

You are the Chief Medical Officer at a community hospital. Your hospital has a small ICU with 10 beds. Based on the results of this study, should you implement the infection control program used in this study?

---

266 Haynes et al. A surgical safety checklist to reduce morbidity and mortality in a global population. NEJM. 2009;360:491-99.

267 de Vries et al. Effect of a comprehensive surgical safety system on patient outcomes. NEJM. 2010 Nov 363;20: 1928-1937.

268 Bouadma et al. Long-term impact of a multifaceted prevention program on ventilator-associated pneumonia in a medical intensive care unit. Clin Infect Dis. 2010;51(10):1115.

269 Berenholtz et al. Collaborative cohort study of an intervention to reduce ventilator-associated pneumonia in the intensive care unit. Infect Control Hosp Epidemiol. 2011;32(4):305.

SUGGESTED ANSWER:

This study suggests that implementation of a safety initiative involving 5 simple infection-control measures by ICU staff was associated with a substantial reduction in catheter-related blood stream infections. However, implementation of a similar program at your hospital will require an investment of staff time and resources. In addition, the program may not work as effectively at your hospital as it did in the Michigan hospitals involved in this study.

As the Chief Medical Officer, you must decide whether the investment is worth it or whether the resources could be used in better ways (e.g. to hire more clinical staff). Many experts believe that implementation of the safety initiative used in this study would be a good investment since the program is relatively inexpensive and seems to substantially reduce infections – which are not only harmful to patients but also expensive to treat. However, as Chief Medical Officer you must ultimately make this decision based on your judgment.

EARLY PALLIATIVE CARE IN NON-SMALL-CELL LUNG CANCER[270]

"Early integration of palliative care with standard oncologic care in patients with metastatic non-small-cell lung cancer resulted in survival that was prolonged by approximately 2 months and clinically meaningful improvements in quality of life and mood."

- Temel et al.[270]

Research Question: Can early palliative care improve the quality of life of patients with metastatic non-small-cell lung cancer (NSCLC)? Also, what is the impact of early palliative care on survival?

Funding: An American Society of Clinical Oncology Career Development Award, as well as gifts from two cancer foundations.

Year Study Began: 2006

---

270 Ternel et al. Early palliative care for patients with metastatic non-small-cell lung cancer. N Engl J Med. 2010 Aug 19;363(8):733-42.

Year Study Published: 2010

Study Location: Massachusetts General Hospital, Boston, Massachusetts

Who Was Studied: Patients in the ambulatory care setting with metastatic NSCLC diagnosed within the previous 8 weeks. In addition, patients were required to have an Eastern Cooperative Oncology Group performance status of 0, 1, or 2 (0=asymptomatic; 1=symptomatic but fully ambulatory; and 2=symptomatic and in bed <50% of the day).

Who Was Excluded: Patients who were already receiving palliative care services.

How Many Patients: 151

Study Overview:

Figure 1: Summary of the Trial's Design

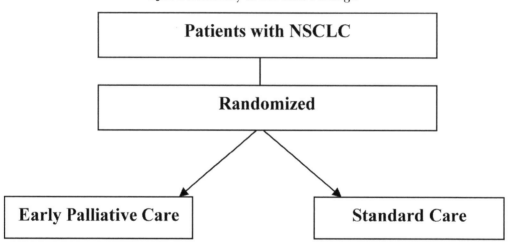

Study Intervention: Patients in the early palliative care group met with a palliative care physician or nurse within three weeks of enrollment and at least monthly thereafter. Additional palliative care visits could be scheduled as needed. The palliative care visits focused on assessing emotional and physical symptoms, establishing goals of care, and coordinating care.

Patients in the standard care group received palliative care visits only when meetings were requested by the patient, the family, or the oncologist.

Patients in both groups received standard cancer therapy throughout the study.

Follow-Up: 12 weeks for the primary analysis, over a year for the survival analysis

Endpoints: Primary outcome: Change from baseline to 12 weeks in quality of life scores, which were measured using components of the Functional

Assessment of Cancer Therapy-Lung (FACT-L) scale. The components of the scale that were used included physical and functional well-being, as well as "seven symptoms specific to lung cancer." Secondary outcomes: Depression, as assessed by the Hospital Anxiety and Depression scale and the Patient Health Questionnaire 9; health care utilization; documentation of resuscitation preferences; and survival.

RESULTS:

- patients in the early palliative care group received an average of 4 palliative care visits

- 14% of patients in the standard care group received a palliative care consultation during the first 12 weeks of the study

Table 1: Summary of the Trial's Key Findings

Outcome	Early Palliative Care Group	Standard Care Group	P Value
Change in quality of life scores[a]	+2.3	-2.3	0.04
Symptoms of Depression[b]	16%	38%	0.01
Aggressive end-of-life care[c]	33%	54%	0.05
Documentation of resuscitation preferences	53%	28%	0.05
Median Survival	11.6 months	8.9 months	0.02

[a]Scores on the scale range from 0 to 84 with higher scores indicating a better quality of life. At baseline, the mean score in the early palliative care group was 56.2 vs. 55.3 in the standard care group.
[b]As assessed using the Hospital Anxiety and Depression Scale. A similar pattern was seen when depression was assessed using the Patient Health Questionnaire 9.
[c]The authors classified patients as having received aggressive end-of-life care if they received chemotherapy within 14 days of death, did not receive hospice care, or were admitted to hospice within 3 days of death.

Criticisms and Limitations: It is not clear whether the benefits of early palliative care resulted from particular components of the intervention, or whether the benefits resulted from additional time and attention from the palliative care team.

Other Relevant Studies and Information:

- The ENABLE II trial showed that a palliative care intervention in patients with advanced cancer led to improvements in quality of life and mood, but not to improvements in symptom intensity or a reduction in hospital or emergency room visits[271]. A post-hoc analysis did not show a significant effect of the intervention on survival (median survival was 14 months in the palliative care group vs. 8.5 months for the standard care group, P=0.14)[271]. The ENABLE II intervention was largely telephone-based.

SUMMARY AND IMPLICATIONS:

Palliative care consultation soon after the diagosis of NSCLC not only has beneficial effects on quality of life and symptoms of depression, but it also appears to prolong survival. Early palliative care is an appropriate component of standard therapy for NSCLC and perhaps other advanced cancers.

CLINICAL CASE: EARLY PALLIATIVE CARE CONSULTATION

CASE HISTORY:

A 74 year old woman is diagnosed with metastatic ovarian cancer. She is seen in your oncology clinic for an initial consultation two weeks later. In addition to discussing her therapeutic options, should you refer this patient for a palliative care consultation?

---

271 Bakitas et al. Effects of a palliative care intervention on clinical outcomes in patients with advanced cancer: the Project ENABLE II randomized controlled trial. JAMA. 2009 Aug 19;302(7):741-9.

SUGGESTED ANSWER:

Although this trial only involved patients with NSCLC, it demonstrated the value of palliative care services in improving quality of life and symptoms of depression in patients with advanced cancer. In addition, early palliative care consultation was associated with prolonged survival.

Metastatic ovarian cancer, like metastatic NSCLC, has a poor prognosis: patients with stage III or IV ovarian cancer have a 5-year survival rate of less than 50%. While no well-designed trials have evaluated the impact of early palliative care among patients with metastatic ovarian cancer, based on the results of this trial it is likely that early palliative care is beneficial. Thus, it would be quite appropriate to refer this patient to a palliative care specialist who could help manage your patient's emotional and physical symptoms and could help to establish realistic goals of care. (Note that palliative care is not synonymous with hospice. Hospice is designed for patients at the end of life whose primary goal is comfort rather than extending life. Palliative care is designed to improve quality of life among patients with serious illnesses who frequently are receiving therapy aimed at extending – or curing – a disease.)

DIRECTLY OBSERVED THERAPY FOR THE TREATMENT OF TUBERCULOSIS IN BALTIMORE[272]

"[Since] implementing community-based [directly observed therapy], Baltimore's annual [tuberculosis] case rates dropped the most, both in absolute and relative terms, compared with the other major cities in this study."

- Chaulk et al.[272]

Research Question: Is directly observed therapy (DOT) effective in lowering the rates of tuberculosis (TB) in communities?

Funding: This was an unfunded analysis using publicly available data.

Year Study Began: 1981

---

272 Chaulk et al. Eleven years of community-based directly observed therapy for tuberculosis. JAMA. 1995;274:945-951.

Year Study Published: 1995

Study Location: Baltimore, Maryland

Study Overview: This study evaluated trends in TB rates in the 11-year period after introduction of a community-based DOT program in Baltimore in 1981. Trends in TB rates were compared between Baltimore and the five major U.S. cities with the highest TB rates but which did not have citywide DOT programs (Miami, San Francisco, Newark, Atlanta, and Washington, DC).

In addition, TB rates were compared between Baltimore and the 19 major U.S. cities with the highest TB rates. Some of these 19 cities had DOT programs, though most programs were not as comprehensive as Baltimore's[273].

Study Intervention: In 1981, the Baltimore city health department began a citywide program in which patients with newly diagnosed TB were offered DOT. Participating patients were assigned to a case management team (each with caseloads of 25-35 patients) which provided direct observation of patients taking their medications (DOT). Prior to hospital discharge, a member of the team (a public health nurse) visited patients to explain the program and to link patients to other public services that they might benefit from. Patients were given the option to receive DOT in several different locations such as the home, work place, school, or local clinic, and approximately 90% of patients opted to receive DOT within their own community (e.g. in their own home).

As part of the program, patients received standard anti-TB medications, which were free to the patient and were administered 5 days a week for the first 15-60 days of therapy and then twice-weekly for the remainder of the treatment course. Patients who frequently missed appointments were aggressively pursued by the case management team.

Patients who opted not to participate in the DOT program received treatment from private physicians.

Follow-Up: 11 years

Endpoints: TB case rates, three-month sputum conversion rates (i.e. the rate of negative sputum cultures after three months of therapy for patients with culture-positive TB), and the rate of therapy completion.

---

273 Chaulk CP and Kajandjian VA. Directly observed therapy for treatment completion of pulmonary tuberculosis: Consensus Statement of the Public Health Tuberculosis Guidelines Panel. JAMA. 1998 Mar 25;279(12):943-8.

RESULTS:

- during the third year of the program, 54% of patients with TB in Baltimore participated in the DOT program, while in the 11th year 76% participated

- patients from Baltimore who agreed to participate in DOT had higher 3-month sputum conversion rates that did patients who opted not to participate; for example, in the final year of the study sputum conversion rates were 86.8% among DOT patients vs. 38.5% among privately treated patients

- three-month sputum conversion rates were higher in Baltimore (76.1%, including both patients who did and did not participate in DOT) than in any of the five comparison cities without comprehensive DOT

- therapy completion rates were higher in Baltimore (78.1%, including both patients who did and did not participate in DOT) than in any of the five comparison cities without comprehensive DOT except for San Francisco (84.6%)

- Baltimore had the 6th highest TB rate among U.S. cities at the beginning of the study vs. the 28th highest at the end

Table 1: Trends in TB Case Rates, 1981-1992[a]

Group	1981	1992	Percentage Change[b]
Baltimore	35.6	17.2	-51.7%
5 Cities with Highest TB Rates without Citywide DOT	52.4	53.5	+2.1%
20 Cities with Highest TB Rates[c]	34.1	33.6	+1.8%[d]

[a]Rates are per 100,000 persons.
[b]No statistical testing reported.
[c]Includes Baltimore along with the 19 other cities with the highest TB rates.
[d]Includes the 19 cities with the highest TB rates besides Baltimore.

Criticisms and Limitations: It is possible that Baltimore's success in managing TB resulted not from the DOT program but rather from other factors. For example, if immigration rates in Baltimore were lower than in other cities, this could lead to a reduction in TB cases in Baltimore. However, the author's analysis did not seem to suggest that other factors – such as rates of AIDS, immigration, poverty, or unemployment – explained Baltimore's success.

Other Relevant Studies and Information:

- DOT presumably leads to a reduction in tuberculosis rates in a population because patients are treated more effectively and are thus less likely to spread the disease to others.

- Other DOT programs, both community-wide programs and those targeted at patients at high risk for relapse, have also been shown to be beneficial[274]. In addition, some studies have suggested that DOT may reduce the rates of drug-resistant tuberculosis[275]

- Several analyses, including some based on the Baltimore experience, have suggested that although DOT is expensive, it is cost-effective[276,277,278]. The savings from DOT result from the reduction in TB incidence (leading to fewer patients in need of treatment), the high treatment success rate (leading to a reduction in the need for repeat treatment), and the likely reduction in multi-drug resistant TB (which is extremely expensive to treat).

- As part of the Baltimore DOT program, close contacts of patients with TB as well as those with a positive tuberculin-skin test were eligible to receive directly observed preventive therapy (e.g. 6-12 months of isoniazid prophylaxis). It is possible that some of the observed reduction in TB rates during the study period resulted from this component of the program.

- The Centers for Disease Control and the American Thoracic Society recommend that all patients with tuberculosis be offered DOT[279].

---

274 Hill AR, Manikal VM, Riska PF. Effectiveness of directly observed therapy (DOT) for tuberculosis: a review of multinational experience reported in 1990-2000. Medicine (Baltimore) 2002; 81:179.

275 Weis et al. The effect of directly observed therapy on the rates of drug resistance and relapse in tuberculosis. N Engl J Med. 1994;330(17):1179.

276 Chaulk et al. Modeling the epidemiology and economics of directly observed therapy in Baltimore. Int J Tuberc Lung Dis. 2000 Mar;4(3):201-7.

277 Moore et al. Cost-effectiveness of directly observed vs. self-administered therapy for tuberculosis. Am J Respir Crit Care Med. 1996 Oct;154(4 Pt 1):1013-9.

278 Burman WJ, Dalton CB, Cohn DL, Butler JR, Reves RR. A cost-effectiveness analysis of directly observed therapy vs self-administered therapy for treatment of tuberculosis. Chest. 1997 Jul;112(1):63-70.

279 Treatment of tuberculosis. American Thoracic Society, CDC, Infectious Diseases Society of America. MMWR Recomm Rep. 2003;52(RR-11):1.

SUMMARY AND IMPLICATIONS:

Implementation of a citywide community-based DOT program in Baltimore was associated with improved treatment compliance among patients with TB and higher treatment success (as defined by sputum conversion rates). Following implementation, TB rates in Baltimore decreased substantially while TB rates increased slightly in comparison cities. While it is possible that Baltimore's success was unrelated to the DOT program, it appears that community-based DOT leads to lower population rates of TB.

CLINICAL CASE: DIRECTLY OBSERVED THERAPY FOR THE TREATMENT OF TUBERCULOSIS

CASE HISTORY:

You are the Commissioner of Health for your state. Rates of tuberculosis in your state are slightly higher than average for the U.S. You were impressed by the success with DOT for patients with tuberculosis in Baltimore. However, because of a budget shortfall, your resources are limited. Should you invest in DOT for patients with tuberculosis in your state?

SUGGESTED ANSWER:

The study in Baltimore, as well as several other studies, have suggested that DOT leads to a reduction in tuberculosis rates in a population. Implementing DOT is expensive, however, since case managers must be assigned to directly observe patients taking their medications. Still, studies have suggested that DOT is cost-effective in the long run because of the expected reduction in TB incidence (leading to fewer patients in need of treatment), the high treatment success rate (leading to a reduction in need for repeat treatment), and the likely reduction in multi-drug resistant TB (which is extremely expensive to treat). Thus, if at all possible with your limited resources, you should try to offer DOT for all patients with tuberculosis in your state – or at least for those with risk factors for medication non-compliance.

STUDY QUESTIONS

1. The Diabetes Prevention Program demonstrated that:
   a.) Both metformin and lifestyle modifications can prevent or delay the development of diabetes.
   b.) Lifestyle modifications and metformin can prevent diabetes-related complications such as microvascular disease.
   c.) To prevent one case of diabetes over three years, approximately 7 people must be treated with metformin or approximately 14 must be treated with a lifestyle-intervention program.
   d.) To prevent one case of diabetes over three years, approximately 7 people must be treated with a lifestyle-intervention program or approximately 14 must be treated with metformin.

2. The trial evaluating four diets with different compositions of fat, protein, and carbohydrates found that:
   a.) Low fat diets were more effective than the other dieting strategies.
   b.) Low carbohydrate diets were more effective than the other dieting strategies.
   c.) All four diets resulted in modest weight loss over two years. There were no significant differences among the groups.
   d.) None of the four strategies was successful.

3. The Physicians' Health Study and Women's Health Study found that aspirin:
   a.) Leads to a small reduction in the risk of myocardial infarction in apparently healthy men and a small reduction in the risk of stroke in healthy women. Aspirin also decreases bleeding risk in both men and women.
   b.) Leads to a small increase in the risk of myocardial infarction in apparently healthy men and a small increase in the risk of stroke in healthy women. Aspirin also increases bleeding risk in both men and women.
   c.) Has no impact on cardiovascular risk or bleeding risk in either apparently healthy men or women.

d.) Leads to a small reduction in the risk of myocardial infarction in apparently healthy men and a small reduction in the risk of stroke in healthy women. Aspirin also increases bleeding risk in both men and women.

4. The Women's Health Initiative found that:
   a.) The overall risks and benefits of combined hormone therapy cancel each other out.
   b.) Among women with existing heart disease, there was a lower rate of cardiovascular disease among women who took combined hormone therapy.
   c.) Randomized trials are not always accurate.
   d.) The risks (cardiovascular disease and breast cancer) of combined hormone therapy outweigh the benefits (a reduction in fractures). In addition, the WHI demonstrates the importance of randomized trials – rather than observational studies – before new therapies become the standard of care.

5. The ERSPC trial found that screening for prostate cancer with PSA testing every four years:
   a.) Leads to a small reduction in prostate cancer deaths along with a substantial increase in the (potentially unnecessary) diagnosis and treatment of prostate cancer.
   b.) Leads to a substantial reduction in prostate cancer deaths, and has no effect on the rate of prostate cancer diagnosis.
   c.) Has no impact on prostate cancer mortality.
   d.) Leads to a reduction in all-cause mortality.

6. The Cochrane Review of screening mammography found that:
   a.) For every 2000 women offered screening mammograms over a 10-year period, 1 will have her life prolonged while 10 will be treated for breast cancer unnecessarily.
   b.) For every 2000 women offered screening mammograms over a 10-year period, 10 will have their lives prolonged while 1 will be treated for breast cancer unnecessarily.
   c.) Screening mammography clearly leads to an all-cause mortality benefit.
   d.) Screening mammography is substantially more beneficial among women 40-49 than it is among women 50 years and older.

7. The Future II trial found that, among girls and women 15 – 26, the quadrivalent HPV vaccine:
   a.) Led to a reduction in the rates of invasive cervical cancer.

    b.) Led to a modest absolute reduction in high-grade cervical lesions that are precursors to cervical cancer.

    c.) Prevented the development of high-grade cervical lesions due to HPV-16 and HPV-18 among patients already infected with these HPV types.

    d.) Was ineffective in preventing high-grade cervical lesions.

8. The CAST trial found that:

    a.) Anti-arrhythmic medications are effective in preventing cardiac death following a myocardial infarction.

    b.) The anti-arrhythmic medications encainide, flecainide, and morcizine increased cardiac mortality in patients with a recent myocardial infarction.

    c.) Anti-arrhythmic medications are not effective at suppressing cardiac arrhythmias following a myocardial infarction.

    d.) The trial was stopped early, before any conclusive results were available.

9. The ALLHAT trial found that chlorthalidone is:

    a.) Inferior to amlodipine and lisinopril as first-line therapy in high risk patients with hypertension.

    b.) Superior to amlodipine but inferior to lisinopril as first-line therapy in high risk patients with hypertension.

    c.) At least as effective as – and in some respects superior to – amlodipine and lisinopril as first-line therapy in high risk patients with hypertension.

    d.) Superior to hydrochlorothiazide as first-line therapy in high risk patients with hypertension.

10. The JUPITER trial found that statin therapy:

    a.) Does not reduce cardiovascular events in healthy patients with elevated CRP levels and normal lipids.

    b.) Reduced cardiovascular events in healthy patients with elevated CRP levels and normal lipids. The absolute benefits are substantial: just 10 patients must be treated to prevent one cardiovascular event.

    c.) Reduced cardiovascular events in healthy patients with elevated CRP levels and normal lipids, though the absolute benefits of statin therapy were small. The value of CRP testing to assess cardiovascular risk remains uncertain.

    d.) CRP testing clearly and definitively identifies patients who will benefit from statin therapy.

11. The AFFIRM trial found that:
   a.) It is safe to stop anticoagulation in patients with atrial fibrillation who are managed with a strategy of rhythm control.
   b.) In older patients and those with cardiovascular risk factors, a strategy of rate-control is at least as effective as a strategy of rhythm-control in managing atrial fibrillation.
   c.) In older patients and those with cardiovascular risk factors, rhythm-control is superior to rate-control in managing atrial fibrillation.
   d.) In young patients without cardiovascular risk factors, rate-control is at least as effective as rhythm-control in managing atrial fibrillation.

12. The RACE II trial found that:
   a.) A strict heart rate target of <80 beats per minute at rest is more effective than a lenient target of <110 beats per minute in patients with permanent atrial fibrillation.
   b.) A strict heart rate target of <80 beats per minute at rest leads to better symptom control and fewer episodes of heart failure than a lenient target of <110 beats per minute in patients with permanent atrial fibrillation.
   c.) A lenient heart rate target of <110 beats per minute at rest is as effective as a strict target of <80 beats per minute in patients with permanent atrial fibrillation.
   d.) The majority of patients with atrial fibrillation do not require any medications.

13. The MERIT-HF trial demonstrated that, in patients with chronic systolic heart failure, metoprolol CR/XL:
   a.) Was poorly tolerated and led to a high rate of syncope.
   b.) Increased mortality, increased hospitalizations, and worsened symptoms and quality of life.
   c.) Reduced mortality, but increased hospitalizations, and worsened symptoms and quality of life.
   d.) Reduced mortality, prevented hospitalizations, and improved symptoms and quality of life.

14. The COURAGE trial showed that for patients with stable coronary artery disease:
   a.) Percutaneous coronary intervention (PCI) leads to increased mortality compared with medical therapy.
   b.) Percutaneous coronary intervention (PCI) leads to decreased mortality compared medical therapy.

c.) Medical therapy and percutaneous coronary intervention (PCI) lead to similar outcomes.

d.) Medical therapy leads to better symptom control but percutaneous coronary intervention (PCI) leads to lower mortality.

15. The ACCORD trial found that a HbA1c target of 6.0% in patients with type 2 diabetes is associated with:
    a.) Decreased mortality compared with a target of 7.0%-7.9%.
    b.) Increased mortality compared with a target of 7.0%-7.9%.
    c.) Fewer hypoglycemic episodes compared with a target of 7.0%-7.9%.
    d.) Less weight gain compared with a target of 7.0%-7.9%.

16. The United Kingdom Prospective Diabetes Study (UKPDS):
    a.) Showed that dietary therapy was as effective as medications for managing patients with type 2 diabetes.
    b.) Was the first study to conclusively show the benefits of medications for treating elevated blood sugar in patients with type 2 diabetes. These benefits persisted 10 years after the trial was stopped.
    c.) Showed that metformin, insulin, and sulfonylureas are effective for preventing the development of type 2 diabetes.
    d.) Metformin is more likely to cause hypoglycemic episodes and weight gain than insulin and sulfonylureas.

17. The African American Heart Failure Trial (A-HeFT) showed that:
    a.) Isosorbide dinitrate/hydralazine is more effective among African Americans with heart failure than among Caucasians with heart failure.
    b.) Isosorbide dinitrate/hydralazine is as effective as angiotensin-converting-enzyme inhibitors for treating African Americans with New York Heart Association class III or IV heart failure and a reduced ejection fraction.
    c.) Isosorbide dinitrate/hydralazine is ineffective in African Americans with New York Heart Association class III or IV heart failure and a reduced ejection fraction.
    d.) Isosorbide dinitrate/hydralazine, when added to standard heart failure therapy, improves outcomes in African Americans with New York Heart Association class III or IV heart failure and a reduced ejection fraction.

18. The NA-ACCORD study of patients with HIV suggests that initiation of antiretroviral therapy in asymptomatic patients who have CD4+ counts of 351-500 as well as counts >500 is:
    a.) Ineffective.

b.) Beneficial. However, since the study was not a randomized trial the results are far from definitive.

c.) Beneficial. This large randomized trial definitively demonstrates the optimal time to initiate antiretroviral therapy.

d.) Harmful.

19. The IDEAL trial found that, with appropriate clinical management, patients with progressive chronic kidney disease:

a.) Can safely delay dialysis initiation until they either develop signs or symptoms indicating the need for dialysis or until their glomerular filtration rate (GFR) drops below 7.0 ml per minute.

b.) Should initiate dialysis when their GFR drops below 15.0 ml per minute.

c.) Can safely delay dialysis initiation until their GFR drops below 7.0 ml per minute even if they develop signs or symptoms indicating the need for dialysis before reaching this threshold.

d.) Should receive hemodialysis rather than peritoneal dialysis whenever possible.

20. The trial of early goal-directed therapy found that:

a.) Patients with severe sepsis or septic shock should be managed with aggressive hemodynamic monitoring and support immediately upon presentation to the emergency room (or, if this is not possible, in the intensive care unit) for 6 hours or until there is resolution of hemodynamic disturbances.

b.) Aggressive hemodynamic monitoring and support is particularly important several hours after patients with sepsis present to the emergency room.

c.) Aggressive hemodynamic management of patients presenting with severe sepsis or septic shock is ineffective and perhaps harmful.

d.) Patients with severe sepsis or septic shock require blood transfusions to keep their hemoglobin above 10.0.

21. The TRICC trial found that for most critically ill patients:

a.) Waiting to transfuse red cells until the hgb drops below 7.0 g/dl leads to worse outcomes than transfusing at a hgb <10.0 g/dl.

b.) Waiting to transfuse red cells until the hemoglobin drops below 7.0 g/dl is at least as effective as, and likely preferable to, transfusing at a hemoglobin <10.0 g/dl.

c.) Waiting to transfuse red cells until the hgb drops below 6.0 g/dl is at least as effective as, and likely preferable to, transfusing at a hgb <10.0 g/dl.

d.) Red cell transfusions are completely unnecessary.

22. The trial of pulmonary artery catheterization in critically ill patients showed that:
   a.) Pulmonary artery catheterization did not lead to improved outcomes compared to standard care without catheterization.
   b.) Pulmonary artery catheterization led to a reduction in the length of stay in the intensive care unit and hospital.
   c.) Pulmonary artery catheterization was superior to standard care without catheterization.
   d.) Many physicians feel it is unethical to withhold pulmonary artery catheterization, and therefore the trial was terminated early.

23. The DIAMOND trial found that:
   a.) For patients with new-onset dyspepsia, a step-up strategy in which patients are first given an antacid, followed by an H2-receptor antagonist, and then a proton pump inhibitor was as effective as a step-down strategy in which a proton pump inhibitor is given first, followed by an H2-receptor antagonist, and then an antacid. The step-up strategy was more cost effective.
   b.) For patients with new-onset dyspepsia, a step-up strategy in which patients are first given an antacid, followed by an H2-receptor antagonist, and then a proton pump inhibitor was superior to a step-down strategy in which a proton pump inhibitor is given first, followed by an H2-receptor antagonist, and then an antacid. The step-down strategy was more cost effective, however.
   c.) For patients with new-onset dyspepsia, a step-down strategy in which a proton pump inhibitor is given first, followed by an H2-receptor antagonist, and then an antacid was superior to a step-up strategy in which patients are first given an antacid, followed by an H2-receptor antagonist, and then a proton pump inhibitor. The step-down strategy was also more cost effective.
   d.) All patients with new-onset dyspepsia should receive H. pylori testing prior to the initiation of any treatment.

24. The trial evaluating opioids in patients with non-cancer related pain demonstrated that, after 11 weeks of treatment, sustained-release oral morphine led to a:
   a.) No improvement in pain or psychological or functional outcomes.
   b.) Modest reduction in pain but no clear improvement in psychological or functional outcomes. Patients in the morphine group experienced a lower rate of gastrointestinal symptoms and dizziness.

c.) High rate of addiction problems.

d.) Modest reduction in pain but no clear improvement in psychological or functional outcomes. Patients in the morphine group experienced an increased rate of gastrointestinal symptoms and dizziness.

25. The POISE trial showed that the initiation of perioperative extended-release metoprolol in patients not currently taking a beta-blocker:

   a.) Lowers the risk of myocardial infarction, stroke, and overall mortality.

   b.) Lowers the risk of myocardial infarction but leads to clinically significant bradycardia and hypotension, and increases the risk of stroke and overall mortality.

   c.) Lowers the risk of stroke but leads to clinically significant bradycardia and hypotension, and increases the risk of myocardial infarction.

   d.) Increases the risk of myocardial infarction, stroke, and overall mortality.

26. The SYNTAX trial found that, for patients with three-vessel and/or left main coronary artery disease:

   a.) Coronary artery bypass grafting (CABG) led to equivalent rates of major cardiovascular and cerebrovascular events compared with percutaneous coronary intervention (PCI), however patients receiving PCI appeared to have a reduced rate of stroke.

   b.) CABG led to increased rates of major cardiovascular and cerebrovascular events compared with PCI. This difference was largely driven by an increase in the need for repeat revascularization procedures among patients receiving CABG, however patients receiving CABG appeared to have a reduced rate of stroke.

   c.) CABG led to reduced rates of major cardiovascular and cerebrovascular events compared with PCI. This difference was largely driven by a reduction in the need for repeat revascularization procedures among patients receiving CABG, however patients receiving PCI appeared to have a reduced rate of stroke.

   d.) CABG and PCI were both inferior to optimal medical therapy.

27. The ACST trial found that in patients with asymptomatic carotid stensosis:

   a.) Surgical management is clearly preferable to medical management.

   b.) Carotid endarterectomy is associated with approximately a 3% perioperative risk, however after several years patients who receive surgery have a lower rate of stroke.

   c.) Medical management is clearly preferable to surgical management in patients with asymptomatic carotid stensosis.

   d.) The perioperative risks of carotid endarterectomy are negligible.

28. The trial of arthroscopic surgery for osteoarthritis of the knee showed that:
    a.) Surgery is superior to management with physical therapy, an individualized exercise program, and pain medications.
    b.) Only patients with mechanical symptoms of catching or locking benefit from surgery.
    c.) Surgery does not appear to offer significant benefits compared to management with physical therapy, an individualized exercise program, and pain medications.
    d.) Trials of surgical interventions are almost always unreliable.

29. The MRC spine stabilization trial suggested that, among patients with chronic low back pain:
    a.) Surgery results in worse pain control compared with non-operative treatment. Patients with chronic low back pain should never receive surgery.
    b.) Surgery may lead to slight improvements in pain control compared with non-operative treatment, however most patients improve substantially without surgery as well. The appropriate role of surgery in patients with chronic low back pain remains uncertain.
    c.) Surgery leads to considerable improvements in pain control compared with non-operative treatment, and all patients with chronic low back pain should receive surgery.
    d.) Pain symptoms worsen considerably over time both among patients treated surgically and among patients treated non-operatively.

30. The B-06 trial comparing mastectomy with breast conserving surgery for women with early stage breast cancer showed that total mastectomy:
    a.) Improves survival compared with breast conserving therapy however total mastectomy is associated with a worse cosmetic result.
    b.) Does not reduce either disease-free survival or overall survival compared with breast conserving therapy. Additionally, breast irradiation following lumpectomy does not reduce the risk of local breast cancer recurrence compared with lumpectomy alone.
    c.) Decreases survival compared with breast conserving surgery.
    d.) Does not reduce either disease-free survival or overall survival compared with breast conserving therapy. Breast irradiation following lumpectomy reduces the risk of local cancer recurrence and leads to a small reduction in breast cancer related mortality, but this reduction is partially offset by an increase in deaths from other causes.

31. The Swedish Obese Subjects Study found that:
    a.) Bariatric surgery reduces the incidence of diabetes, but has no effect on mortality rates.
    b.) Bariatric surgery leads to long-term weight loss and a modest but detectable reduction in all-cause mortality in patients with severe obesity.
    c.) The fatal complication rate from bariatric surgery exceeds 1%.
    d.) Gastric bypass, but not gastric banding or vertical banded gastroplasty, leads to long-term weight loss and a reduction in all-cause mortality in patients with severe obesity.

32. The CMPPT trial showed that in women with post-term (≥41 weeks) pregnancies, induction of labor results in a:
    a.) Large, significant decrease in the rate of perinatal mortality and neonatal morbidity.
    b.) Large increase in the rate of perinatal mortality and neonatal morbidity.
    c.) Slight increase in the rate of cesarean section compared with serial monitoring.
    d.) Slight decrease in the rate of cesarean section compared with serial monitoring.

33. According to the trial evaluating antepartum glucocorticoids in women presenting with premature labor, antenatal betamethasone:
    a.) Is ineffective in preventing respiratory distress syndrome and perinatal mortality in neonates.
    b.) Is effective in preventing respiratory distress syndrome and perinatal mortality in neonates. The treatment is most effective among women experiencing premature labor prior to 32 weeks of gestation and when the betamethasone is given at least 24 hours before delivery.
    c.) Is effective in preventing respiratory distress syndrome and perinatal mortality in neonates. The treatment is most effective among women experiencing premature labor after 32 weeks of gestation.
    d.) Is effective in preventing respiratory distress syndrome and perinatal mortality in neonates. The treatment is most effective when the betamethasone is given within 24 hours of delivery.

34. The trial comparing immediate antibiotics (amoxicillin-clavulanate) vs. placebo in children <2 with acute otitis media found that:
    a.) Antibiotics resulted in faster resolution of symptoms and improved clinical cure rates at the end of therapy but an increased rate of side effects (diarrhea and diaper dermatitis).

b.) There was no difference in response rates but there was an increased rate of side effects with antibiotics (diarrhea and diaper rash).

c.) Antibiotics resulted in faster resolution of symptoms and a decreased rate of side effects (diarrhea and diaper rash).

d.) Antibiotics resulted in slower resolution of symptoms and an increased rate of side effects (diarrhea and diaper rash).

35. The trial comparing early vs. delayed placement of ear tubes in children with otitis media and persistent ear effusion found that:

a.) Children who received early placement of ear tubes had lower rates of persistent ear effusion as well as better developmental outcomes.

b.) Children who received early placement of ear tubes had similar rates of persistent ear effusion and worse developmental outcomes.

c.) Although children who received early placement of ear tubes had lower rates of persistent ear effusion, developmental outcomes were no different in the two groups.

d.) There was a high rate of cross over in the trial, and therefore the results are not reliable.

36. The START trial showed that daily inhaled budesonide:

a.) Has no effect on severe asthma exacerbations in children and adults with recent onset mild persistent asthma. In children 5-15, budesonide was associated with a small but detectable reduction in height during the three year study period.

b.) Reduces severe asthma exacerbations in children and adults with recent onset mild persistent asthma. In children 5-15, budesonide did not lead to a reduction in height during the three year study period.

c.) Reduces severe asthma exacerbations in children and adults with recent onset mild persistent asthma. In children 5-15, budesonide was associated with a small but detectable reduction in height during the three year study period.

d.) Increases severe asthma exacerbations in children and adults with recent onset mild persistent asthma. In children 5-15, budesonide was associated with a small but detectable reduction in height during the three year study period.

37. The MTA trial showed that for children with Attention-Deficit/ Hyperactivity Disorder:

a.) Medication management was superior to behavioral treatment alone. Because medications may have adverse effects, however, the decision about whether or not to initiate medications should take into account family preference.

b.) Medication management was equivalent to behavioral treatment alone.

c.) Combined medication management and behavioral treatment, but not medication management alone, was superior to routine community care.

d.) Behavioral therapy is superior to medications for treating children with ADHD.

38. A large cohort study of Danish children who did and did not receive the Measles, Mumps, and Rubella vaccine:

a.) Did not identify a link between the vaccine and autism or autism-spectrum disorders. In addition, there was no clustering of autism diagnoses at any time interval after vaccination.

b.) Showed a strong link between the vaccine and autism-spectrum disorders, with a clustering of diagnoses 6 months after vaccination.

c.) Did not identify a link between the vaccine and autism or autism-spectrum disorders, however there was a clustering of autism diagnoses 12 months after vaccination

d.) Was invalid because it did not control for differences between vaccinated and unvaccinated children.

39. The trial evaluating magnetic resonance imaging (MRI) of the spine in patients with lower back pain found that spinal MRIs (compared with plain radiographs):

a.) Are reassuring to patients with lower back pain and lead to improved functional outcomes.

b.) Are reassuring to patients with lower back pain and decrease overall health care costs by leading to faster resolution of symptoms.

c.) Are highly effective for differentiating clinically important anatomic spinal abnormalities from incidental findings, helping doctors correctly identify appropriate surgical candidates.

d.) Are reassuring to patients with lower back pain, but they do not lead to improved functional outcomes. In addition, spinal MRIs detect anatomical abnormalities that would otherwise go undiscovered, possibly leading to spinal surgeries of uncertain value.

40. The DIAD study found that:

a.) Patients with diabetes without symptoms of coronary artery disease do not appear to benefit from screening stress tests.

b.) Patients with diabetes without symptoms of coronary artery disease should undergo routine coronary angiography.

c.) Patients with diabetes without symptoms of coronary artery disease always require coronary angiography if they have a positive stress test.

    d.) Patients with diabetes without symptoms of coronary artery disease clearly benefit from screening stress tests.

41. The Christopher study found that:
    a.) A simple protocol involving clinical criteria (the modified Wells criteria), D-dimer testing, and computed tomography can safely and effectively exclude acute pulmonary embolism in patients with a clinical suspicion of this disease.
    b.) A simple protocol involving clinical criteria (the modified Wells criteria), D-dimer testing, and computed tomography was ineffective in identifying patients with a likely pulmonary embolism requiring anticoagulation.
    c.) Ventilation/perfusion scans are more effective than computed tomography for diagnosing pulmonary emboli.
    d.) All patients with suspected pulmonary emboli must be evaluated with computed tomography.

42. The study aimed at deriving and evaluating prediction rules for identifying children at very low risk for clinically-important traumatic brain injuries (ci-TBIs) showed that:
    a.) Children with none of the six predictive features are at very low risk (<0.05%) for ci-TBI and generally do not require computed tomography (CT) scans of the head.
    b.) Children with none of the six predictive features are still at considerable risk for ci-TBI and require CT scans for evaluation.
    c.) Children managed according to the predictive rules have superior outcomes to children managed according to usual care.
    d.) Children managed according to the predictive rules have equivalent outcomes to children managed according to usual care.

43. The ECASS III trial showed that, in patients with an acute ischemic stroke, thrombolysis with alteplase:
    a.) Is efficacious when given up to 4.5 hours after the onset of symptoms, however patients treated within the first 1.5 hours have the best outcomes.
    b.) Is ineffective when given 3-4.5 hours after the onset of symptoms.
    c.) Is more efficacious when given 3 to 4.5 hours after the onset of symptoms than when given within the first three hours.
    d.) Is efficacious when given up to 6 hours after the onset of symptoms, however patients treated within the first 1.5 hours have the best outcomes.

44. The trial evaluating depression treatment in primary care practice found that:
    a.) Initial treatment with psychotherapy is superior to initial pharmacotherapy (nortriptyline).
    b.) Initial treatment with psychotherapy and pharmacotherapy (nortriptyline) were equally efficacious, however clinical improvement was slightly faster with pharmacotherapy.
    c.) Initial treatment with pharmacotherapy (nortriptyline) is superior to initial psychotherapy.
    d.) Neither psychotherapy nor pharmacotherapy (nortriptyline) were effective.

45. According to the trial evaluating treatments for insomnia in the elderly, cognitive-behavior therapy (CBT), medication, and combined CBT plus medication:
    a.) Are all equally effective in both the short and long term.
    b.) All improve symptoms of insomnia more than placebo, however medication appeared to have the best outcomes with long term follow-up.
    c.) Do not improve symptoms of insomnia more than placebo.
    d.) All improve symptoms of insomnia more than placebo, however CBT appeared to have the best outcomes with long term follow-up.

46. The Group Health medical home demonstration suggested that:
    a.) Investment in primary care has the potential to improve healthcare quality and perhaps lower costs.
    b.) The medical home model is superior to other primary care models in all practice settings.
    c.) A focus on patients with chronic illness can greatly reduce healthcare costs.
    d.) The medical home model has the potential to improve healthcare quality, but may lead to reduced satisfaction among clinic staff.

47. The trial evaluating Project RED showed that care coordination at the time of hospital discharge:
    a.) Can substantially reduce repeat emergency room and hospital visits.
    b.) Has no impact on repeat emergency room and hospital visits.
    c.) Increases the chances that patients will follow-up with their primary care doctors after discharge but has no impact on repeat emergency room and hospital visits.
    d.) Decreases the chances that patients will follow-up with their primary care doctors after discharge.

48. The Keystone ICU Project analysis showed that implementation of a safety initiative involving 5 simple infection-control measures by intensive care unit staff was associated with:
    a.) Tremendous dissatisfaction among ICU staff.
    b.) No impact on catheter-related blood stream infections.
    c.) A substantial increase in catheter-related blood stream infections.
    d.) A substantial reduction in catheter-related blood stream infections.

49. The "Early Palliative Care in Non-Small-Cell Lung Cancer" trial found that palliative care consultation soon after the diagnosis of non-small-cell lung cancer:
    a.) Has beneficial effects on quality of life and symptoms of depression, but it appears to shorten survival.
    b.) Not only has beneficial effects on quality of life and symptoms of depression, but it also appears to prolong survival.
    c.) Is not effective for improving quality of life or symptoms of depression, and it appears to shorten survival.
    d.) Is not effective for improving quality of life or symptoms of depression, but it appears to prolong survival.

50. The study of directly observed therapy (DOT) for tuberculosis in Baltimore found that following implementation of a citywide community-based DOT program:
    a.) TB rates decreased substantially. During the same time period, TB rates increased slightly in comparison cities.
    b.) TB rates were unchanged. During the same time period, TB rates were also unchanged in comparison cities.
    c.) TB rates increased substantially. During the same time period, TB rates decreased in comparison cities.
    d.) TB rates decreased substantially. However, these results are difficult to assess because, during the same time period, TB rates also decreased substantially in comparison cities.

ANSWERS

1) **D**	2) **C**	3) **D**	4) **D**	5) **A**
6) **A**	7) **B**	8) **B**	9) **C**	10) **C**
11) **B**	12) **C**	13) **D**	14) **C**	15) **B**
16) **B**	17) **D**	18) **B**	19) **A**	20) **A**
21) **B**	22) **A**	23) **A**	24) **D**	25) **B**
26) **C**	27) **B**	28) **C**	29) **B**	30) **D**
31) **B**	32) **D**	33) **B**	34) **A**	35) **C**
36) **C**	37) **A**	38) **A**	39) **D**	40) **A**
41) **A**	42) **A**	43) **A**	44) **B**	45) **D**
46) **A**	47) **A**	48) **D**	49) **B**	50) **A**